Current Trends of Supercritical Fluid Technology

in Pharmaceutical, Nutraceutical and Food Processing

Industries

Editors:

Ana Rita C. Duarte

Catarina M. M. Duarte

eBooks End User License Agreement

CONTENTS

1. INTRODUCTION

2. PHARMACEUTICAL PROCESSING

3. NUTRACEUTICAL AND FOOD PROCESSING

4. SCALE-UP ISSUES

FOREWORD

Research into the domain of supercritical fluids (SCF) science and technology has been pursued actively for more than twenty years. The first world conference devoted to SCFs and their applications was organised by Michel Perrut, the founder and first president of the International Society for the Advancement of Supercritical Fluids (ISASF) in 1988 in Nice (France). Since then, 9 symposia in this series have been held and numerous others are organised all over the world, testifying to the vigour of this field.

Both fundamental and applied research have provided subjects for an exponentially increasing number of papers in specialised journals. However, quite curiously, textbooks devoted to this area remain rather scarce.

At first, the applications dealt essentially with extraction of natural products. But gradually several other domains appeared: material processing (both organic including polymers and inorganic), hydrothermal oxidation and synthesis, particle design, porous media, biomedical applications, chemical and enzymatic reactions, waste and biomass valorisation processes, new catalysts and hybrid materials, and many more.

Among the industrial sectors, pharmacy, cosmetics and agro-food appear to have a prominent place. Especially, particle formation (submicronic, monodisperse,...) and solid formulation (emulsions, coating, encapsulation,...) have attracted recent, innovative and promising developments.

This book updating the knowledge of supercritical fluid technology in pharmaceutical, nutraceutical and food processing is therefore particularly welcome.

At the university of Lisbon, at the beginning of the 21st century, a group headed by Catarina Duarte has specialised in nutraceuticals and related areas and became progressively one of the reference teams in this area. With the help of a former student of hers, Ana Rita Duarte, now working at the university of Minho, they took the excellent initiative to edit this new book. All the contributors of the 10 chapters are renowned specialists in their respective fields and these chapters encompass both the scientific and engineering issues.

There is little doubt that this book will rapidly become essential for both students and researchers willing to remain at the very front line of scientific progress in the fast moving area of supercritical fluid science and technology.

Jacques Fages, Professor,

ISASF President,
RAPSODEE Research Centre
Ecole des Mines,
Albi, France

PREFACE

With world-wide concern for environmental issues, there is a growing opportunity for the utilisation of supercritical fluid (SCF) technologies as green alternatives to conventional processes currently used in the pharmaceutical, cosmetic and food industries.

The application of supercritical fluids as an alternative to conventional precipitation and extraction processes has been an active field of research and innovation during the past decades. The main motivation for this has been the possibility of exploiting the peculiar properties of supercritical fluids, which are often described as intermediate between those of a liquid and a gas, easily changeable with small modifications in operating conditions, namely pressure and temperature. In the case of carbon dioxide (the most used supercritical solvent), the supercritical region can be achieved at moderate conditions of pressure and tempreature, avoiding the degradation of thermolabile substances and providing simultaneously an inert medium suitable for processing easily oxidable compounds. Moreover, the use of the supercritical fluid eliminates or reduces the use of toxic or contaminant organic solvents and the elimination of the supercritical fluid from the final product can be easily accomplished by a simple depressurization.

It has become evident that the identification synthesis or isolation of active components is not sufficient to ensure progress in drug therapy. Considerable effort has been devoted to the development of novel approaches for the delivery and administration of organic active agents. Particle and delivery systems design are major developments of supercritical fluids applications. Because of their high diffusivity, high solvent power and low viscosity, SCFs can be used as solvents or antisolvents to micronize bioactive compounds and bioerodible polymers, and impregnate or encapsulate drugs in biocompatible matrices (natural or synthetic polymers, waxes and fats). The continuous formation of solids following the rapid expansion of a highly compressible supercritical solution is an interesting alternative to conventional crystallization methods used in the pharmaceutical industry (spray-drying, jet milling and grinding). Through the rapid expansion process, a dramatic change of the solute supersaturation is created causing subsequente precipitation of small particles with a narrow size distribution. Also the possibility of using supercritical fluid technology for the formation of composite micro/nano-spheres/capsules and impregnation of different polymers has been explored by various researchers for a number of years now.

Supercritical fluid extraction (SFE) has being explored for production of ever-widening ranges of concentrated natural extracts, with positive physiological activity. In fact, the concern on health care created a major opportunity market for natural products with specific health effects and there has been considerable interest in the last decade in switching from synthetic to natural substances in the food and pharmaceutical industries.

This book aims to contribute to disseminate knowledge related with the application of supercritical fluid technology in the development of "clean" separation processes and preparation of delivery devices, with applications in the pharmaceutical and other emergent industries (such as the nutraceutical and cosmeceutical).

We would like to express our gratitude to the authors of each chapter, without whom this publication wouldn't be possible.

Ana Rita C. Duarte

Catarina M. M. Duarte

CONTRIBUTORS

A. Martín	High Pressure Processes Group. Department of Chemical Engineering and Environmental Technology, University of Valladolid, Spain
A. R. C. Duarte	Researcher, 3B's Research Group, Department of Polymer Engineering, University of Minho, Portugal
	IBB – Institute for Biotechnology and Bioengineering, PT Associated Laboratory (Laboratório Associado), Portugal
A. R. S. de Sousa	Instituto de Tecnologia Química e Biológica, Universidade Nova de Lisboa, Portugal
	Instituto de Biologia Experimental e Tecnológica, Avenida da República, Portugal
C. M. M. Duarte	Instituto de Tecnologia Química e Biológica, Universidade Nova de Lisboa, Portugal
	Instituto de Biologia Experimental e Tecnológica, Portugal
C.J. Peters	The Petroleum Institute, Chemical Engineering Department, Abu Dhabi, United Arab Emirates
E. Kühne	Fluid Flow and Flow Assurance, Shell Global Solutions International B.V., The Netherlands
E. Reverchon	Università degli Studi di Salerno, Dipartimento di Ingegneria Chimica e Alimentare, Italy
F. Deschamps	Separex, France
F. Lebouef	Separex, France
G.J. Witkamp	Laboratory for Process Equipment, Delft University of Technology - Faculty of Mechanical, Maritime and Materials Engineering, The Netherlands
H. Sovova	Institute of Chemical Process Fundamentals of the ASCR, Czech Republic
I. de Marco	Università degli Studi di Salerno, Dipartimento di Ingegneria Chimica e Alimentare, Italy
J. B. Grey	Industrial Research Limited, New Zealand
M. J. Cocero	High Pressure Processes Group. Department of Chemical Engineering and Environmental Technology, University of Valladolid, Spain
N. E. Durling	Industrial Research Limited, New Zealand
O. J. Catchpole	Industrial Research Limited, New Zealand
S. J. Tallon	Industrial Research Limited, New Zealand
W. Eltringham	Industrial Research Limited, New Zealand

CHAPTER 1

Introduction to Supercritical Fluids: Basic Principles and Applications

M. Nunes da Ponte

REQUIMTE, Dep. Chemistry, Faculdade de Ciências e Tecnologia, Universidade Nova de Lisboa, 2829-516 Caparica, Portugal; Email: mnp@dq.fct.unl.pt)

Abstract: This paper provides a short overview of developments in the field of supercritical fluids in the last thirty yearsand of actual and prospective applications

THE BEGINNINGS

The 1978 Symposium on Supercritical Extraction held in Essen, Germany [1], brought the developments of supercritical technology achieved mostly in Germany during the 1970s to the attention of the Chemical and Process Engineering world research community.

The same year, the coffee company Kaffee HAG inaugurated in Bremen its new decaffeination plant, the first high tonnage commercial application of supercritical carbon dioxide. These two events marked the beginning of the thirty years of continuous attention that supercritical fluids have been enjoying.

Of course, the vapour-liquid critical point and the main features of supercritical fluids had been known since the 19th century, and related to such well-known scientists as Andrews and van der Waals. The ICI process for production of polyethylene, discovered in the early 20th century, is still, arguably, the highest tonnage application of supercritical fluid technology. In fact, in this process, high pressure ethylene is simultaneously reactant and supercritical solvent. More recently, the ROSE (Residual Oil Supercritical Extraction) process, which uses supercritical propane, was developed by the petrochemical industry, and it is often cited as an early application.

However, the supercritical fluid image that emerged from the Essen Symposium had a different and special appeal. It was based on supercritical carbon dioxide as a natural, innocuous, easy-to-separate solvent that might replace volatile organic solvents, which were just starting to be universally perceived as harmful pollutants. This image brought into the field researchers from a wide array of disciplines, also an important factor in subsequent developments.

The books of McHugh and Krukonis [2] and of Stahl, Quirin and Gerard [3] were among the first to summarise the quickly increasing literature already available in the mid-eighties. Since then, the field of supercritical fluids diversified from the initial focus on extraction with carbon dioxide into many areas.

One major development was the appearance of water as a second focus of attention of the supercritical fluid community. Although the commercial use of supercritical water has been hampered by the extreme conditions of its use, water has had a strong appeal as the natural supercritical solvent *par excellence*.

In the last thirty years, a wide range of fundamental studies were published and many patents were submitted, with potential applications in separation processes, chemistry, materials. Many books and reviews were published on different aspects of supercritical fluids. In recent years, the Journal of Supercritical Fluids has consistently been ranked as one of the top ten journals of Chemical Engineering in terms of citation-based impact factors. This journal has recently published a commemorative issue of its 20th anniversary, consisting of 33 articles, which comprehensively review the field [4].

SUPERCRITICAL FLUIDS AND THEIR PROPERTIES

Supercritical fluids are often referred as existing in a state somewhat between gases and liquids. In fact they are gases at pressure and temperatures above (but not much) those of the vapour-liquid critical point. As the critical pressures of known substances are (much) higher than atmospheric pressure, a first consequence is that a supercritical fluid is always a high pressure gas, and using them requires high pressure technology.

The really unique property of supercritical fluids is their ability to respond to small changes in pressure or temperature with large variations of density, without undergoing a phase change. Density is directly related to many other physical and chemical properties of a fluid. The most important in many supercritical fluid applications is solvent power, that is, the ability to dissolve other substances. With small relative changes in pressure (or temperature), a supercritical fluid can be brought from relatively low density, where it can hardly dissolve anything, to liquid-like densities, where the molecules of the fluid can cluster around the molecules of solid or liquid solutes and bring them into the gas phase.

A good example is given by carbon dioxide, typically used in many applications at a temperature of about 50 °C and pressures above 10 MPa. According to the correlation of Span et al. [5], the density doubles between 10 and 19 MPa, from around 0.4 kg dm^{-3} to close to 0.8 kg dm^{-3}, a density typical of organic liquid solvents. Carbon dioxide, as any other supercritical gas, can therefore be used as if it were two or even several solvents, in a pressure or temperature-dependent way.

Most applications of supercritical fluids are developed around a higher pressure compartment or vessel and a lower pressure one. In the first, the supercritical solvent promotes dissolution/extraction/reaction or any other intended higher density-dependent effect. In the second one, decompression often leads to separation of products from the fluid.

In the case of water, its properties as a solvent vary considerably as temperature increases, due to the gradual disruption of its three-dimension hydrogen bond network, which starts to occur well below the critical temperature (374 °C). At high temperatures, water behaves as a highly polar "non-aqueous" solvent, dissolving hydrocarbons and precipitating ionic salts. It is also a highly reactive medium, promoting a variety of chemical reactions, as exemplified by the importance of hot, pressurised aqueous solutions (the so-called hydrothermal fluids) in geochemical processes.

One important property of water is the ionic product K_w, which increases with temperature and density. At 1000 °C and liquid-like densities, K_w is around six orders of magnitude larger than at room temperature. Weingartner and Franck [6] point out that this change has a high impact on hydrolysis and acid–base equilibrium. They give the example of the equilibrium constant of the hydrolysis reaction:

$Cl^- + H_2O \leftrightarrow HCl + OH^-$, which, at 773 K and 200 MPa, is about nine orders of magnitude larger than at normal conditions. This greatly enhances corrosion of the materials of piping and reactors, and the search for new applications of near-critical and supercritical water has been accompanied by the search for new resistant materials. Important advances have been fostered by developments in the energy industrial sector, where supercritical water has been used by newly designed coal-fired power plants, in order to maximize thermodynamic efficiency. In fact, turbine cycles using steam at very high pressure and temperature (actually, water at supercritical conditions) are becoming a new industry standard.

EXTRACTION WITH CARBON DIOXIDE

Extraction with carbon dioxide has been the most important application of supercritical fluids. The advantages of carbon dioxide as solvent in processes involving products for human consumption are well known: it is, in fact, classified as GRAS – generally regarded as safe, it has low toxicity (threshold limit value – TLV = 5000 ppm), and it becomes supercritical just above ambient temperature (critical temperature 31 °C), an important feature when dealing with heat-sensitive substances. It is cheaper than most organic solvents, and, like other supercritical fluids, it has advantageous gas-like transport properties, such as lower viscosity and higher diffusivity than liquid solvents.

Carbon dioxide is a polar substance, because it possesses a permanent quadrupole – an asymmetry of charge distribution where negative charge is pulled towards the outer oxygen atoms, and the carbon atom becomes positive. However it dissolves mostly low molecular weight, non-polar compounds. It is a poor solvent for many other molecules, with some notable exceptions, like perfluorinated ones [7]. This makes extractions and fractionations using carbon dioxide very selective processes, although they can only be used for the few substances that CO_2 can dissolve in reasonable amounts.

Supercritical carbon dioxide extraction of natural products from solid plant matrices is currently an established, mature application, with over one hundred industrial facilities of various sizes operating throughout the world. Several books have been published about it [8].

Although proposed as a "green" process for the replacement of volatile organic solvents, its implementation resulted in each case from definite technological advantages. A perfect example is given by a recently built industrial facility for the extraction of the substance trichloroanisol (TCA) from cork powder with supercritical carbon dioxide. The unit is operating in Spain, and it was described in detail by Lack [9].

TCA is produced by naturally-ocurring fungi and it is a powerful contaminant of cork stoppers for wine bottles. It is the main contributor to the cork taint of wines, which confers a mouldy smell/taste and may completely ruin the whole content of a bottle. Cork is the bark of a tree that finds its habitat in southern Iberia and in other Mediterranean regions. It is a renewable natural product that slowly grows around a tree, until it reaches the required size after nine years. It is then cut out from the tree, which immediately starts growing another protective layer of bark.

Cork is very important for the economy of the rural communities of Southern Iberia, but its main application, wine stoppers, has been under threat from competition of plastic stoppers and screw-caps. One of the main reasons has been the relatively high incidence of cork taint.

Cork is also a special material, where liquid solvents almost do not penetrate. It is therefore not easily amenable to inside cleaning. The above mentioned facility uses the Diamond process, jointly developed by the Centre d'Énergie Atomique at Pierrelatte and the French cork company Sabaté. It extracts the contaminant trichloroanisol from cork powder with supercritical carbon dioxide.

The selectivity of such a weak solvent as carbon dioxide is used in this process to a big advantage. At moderate pressures, not very far above critical, the solubilities may be finely tuned. The volatile trichloroanisol is soluble in CO_2 and extractable, contrarily to most of the natural constituents of cork. It can therefore be removed from cork without affecting its fundamental properties as a unique material. Moreover, the high diffusivity of CO_2 allows it to penetrate the elaborate cell structure of cork, an effect that cannot be obtained with liquid solvents. Finally, the bactericidal and fungicidal properties of carbon dioxide reduce the microbial load of cork, and prevent further contamination. All these form a unique combination, resulting in a technological advantage that could not be matched until now by any other process.

Another important conclusion of the commercial implementation of this process is that, contrarily to conventional wisdom, the application of supercritical carbon dioxide extraction is not limited to high value-added products. Cork stoppers are cheap, but sold by the millions. Wherever economies of scale are appropriately reached, the cost is not the problem.

Most extraction applications are focused on natural products for human consumption, where the GRAS status of carbon dioxide represents a clear benefit. However other uses have also become commercial, like cleaning of mechanical precision parts or dry-cleaning of clothes. Dry-cleaning is a special case, because it requires the solubilisation of many substances that are essentially insoluble in carbon dioxide. It uses fluorinated surfactants, which are highly soluble in CO_2 and can act as solubility enhancers for many types of molecules.

The cleaning of silicon wafers in the microprocessor industry is a potential high value application. This subject was reviewed by Beckman [10]. He calls attention to its very high potential "green" character, as its implementation would avoid the huge quantities of contaminated cleaning waters that are presently used. One of the technical advantages of the use of carbon dioxide is the drastic reduction of the interfacial tensions, which allows the cleaning of extremely thin crevices, without damaging the structure of the devices.

Fractionation of liquid mixtures with supercritical carbon dioxide in countercurrent columns is a process of the same family of extraction. However, as the raw-materials are liquid, all the intervening substances are fluid, and fractionation is therefore a truly continuous process. This represents a big advantage over extraction from solids, which is usually carried out in batch mode, or at best, like for the decaffeination of coffee beans, in a semi-continuous fashion.

Fractionation with high pressure carbon dioxide may be ideal for difficult separations in liquid mixtures. It has been proposed for separations of valuable substances from natural products, like vegetable food oils, fish oils, wine and beer. The deterpenation of citrus oils is an example of a very difficult separation that has found commercial application. Brunner's book [8] describes fundamentals and design techniques in great detail.

Impregnation may be viewed as the opposite operation to extraction. The use of high pressure carbon dioxide as carrier solvent of substances that deposit inside a material, upon decompression of the solvent, has been proposed in a variety of situations. Although most of these proposals involve plastics and polymers, the best example of the commercialisation of this process may be the production of Superwood, a trademark of the company Supertrae. As reported by Iversen et al. [11], the "world's first supercritical wood treatment plant" was inaugurated in Hampen, Denmark, in 2002. It uses supercritical CO_2 as the carrier solvent of a fungicide that protects the wood from rotting. During decompression in large high pressure vessels of 8 m^3 capacity filled with wooden blocks, the fungicide precipitates and impregnates the wood. The plant has an annual treatment capacity of 40 to 60x10^3 m^3 of wood.

CHEMISTRY IN SUPERCRITICAL SOLVENTS

Supercritical fluids have been used in commercial applications as solvents for chemical reaction since the 1930s in the ICI process for polyethylene, as described above. Their study in the new context of Green Chemistry and clean processes is, however, recent, and developed after the initial focus on extraction. Research on supercritical carbon dioxide and supercritical water as reaction media took off during the 1990s. An overview of the field, edited by Noyori [12], appeared in 1999 in a full issue of Chemical Reviews, comprising 12 separate review papers. Jessop and Leitner's book [13] has also provided a thorough account of the activities in the field, at about the same time.

Supercritical Carbon Dioxide

One of the advantages of using a supercritical fluid as reaction medium is the possibility to integrate reaction and separation, whereby reaction is carried out at high pressure (high density of the solvent) and separation obtained by decompression. Another important advantage is that supercritical fluids mix in all proportions (in principle) with other gases, thus providing the possibility to carry out in a single phase processes that are ordinarily biphasic, like hydrogenation, oxidation with air, hydroformylation.

In the case of CO_2, the fact that it is inert to oxidation and free radical chemistry makes it a desirable solvent for oxidation and free-radical polymerisation reactions. The discovery of DeSimone's group [7] that addition of fluorinated tails to otherwise conventional homogeneous catalysts could increase their solubility in supercritical carbon dioxide greatly improved the possibilities of carrying out homogeneous catalysis in that solvent.

One of the most conspicuous industrial applications of carbon dioxide as reaction medium resulted from the collaboration of Poliakoff's group at Nottingham University and Thomas Swan, a speciality chemicals company [14]. In 2002, Thomas Swan launched what is described in their website as "the world's first continuous phase, high pressure supercritical fluid reactor for both pilot and commercial scale production". The plant had been commissioned to Chematur Engineering Ltd in 1999.

The research work focused on heterogeneous catalysis and hydrogenation, Friedel-Crafts alkylation, etherification and hydroformylation. The hydrogenation of isophorone was the first commercial process to be carried out. The main "green" advantage of this process was that quantitative conversion to the desired product could be achieved, which eliminated the need for downstream separation by energy-intensive distillation [15].

This collaboration earned the Industrial Innovation Team Award of the Industrial Affairs Division of the Royal Society of Chemistry for the work on "developing production scale chemistry in supercritical carbon dioxide".

Another important application of carbon dioxide as reaction solvent that reached the commercial stage resulted from research collaboration between DuPont and the group of DeSimone, at the University of North Carolina. The process produces new grades of poly-tetrafluoroethylene, with supercritical carbon dioxide replacing water as solvent [16].

Supercritical Water

Many interesting reactions were studied in supercritical water. As mentioned above, water in these conditions is a highly reactive substance, and it can act as solvent, reactant and/or catalyst. Hydrolysis, oxidation and pyrolysis of organic compounds have probably been the most studied reactions.

Perhaps the best-known application is SCWO - supercritical water oxidation, which may lead to the total oxidation of organic waste. This process makes use of the increased solubility of most organic compounds in water in supercritical conditions, and of total miscibility with oxygen, to carry out rapid and complete oxidation of waste, producing essentially carbon dioxide, water, and some other small molecules. Many demonstration facilities have been built in recent years to show the feasibility of these methods for waste destruction at large scale. However, the problems of corrosion have not been completely solved yet. Another problem is the deposition of salts, due to the reduction of the dielectric constant of water at low densities.

As any other supercritical fluid, supercritical water has properties that can be fine-tuned by temperature or pressure. Temperatures and pressures may be chosen so that only partial oxidation of organic molecules will occur. The change of the dielectric constant of water with density can also be used to favor the formation of either polar or non-polar oxidation products.

In a recent special issue of the Journal of Supercritical Fluids, hydrolytic [17] and oxidative [18] processes, biomass gasification [19], catalysis [20], and hydrothermal flames [21] in supercritical water are reviewed in separate papers.

The formation of nanoparticles of inorganic substances [22] and the deposition of metals from different compounds [23] have been extensively studied in supercritical water, as well as in supercritical carbon dioxide.

Until now, none of the proposed applications of supercritical water has been used at large scale on a regular basis. But the attractiveness of using water, the ultimate green solvent, for the design of sustainable processes will certainly bring to commercial exploitation many of the current research themes in this area.

EXPANDED LIQUIDS

Carbon dioxide is a relatively poor solvent, but it usually dissolves in large amounts in many organic liquid solvents. The dissolution is often accompanied by considerable expansions in the total volume of the liquid, which can be very sensitive to pressure close to the critical line of the mixture, and reach values of up to 10 times the original volume. The properties of these "expanded" solvents are substantially different from those of the original liquid solvent. Viscosity, interfacial tension and diffusivity are affected, with beneficial effects on mass-transfer. Changes in solubility can be drastic – there is a general decrease of solvent power, with the exception of gaseous solutes, which may dissolve better in the expanded liquid than in the original one. The use of these solvents has been viewed as remedy to the limited usefulness of supercritical carbon dioxide as medium for Chemistry, due to its relatively low capacity as a solvent. In fact, gas-expanded solvents cover a much wider range of solvent power, and they still retain some of the tunability of properties with pressure (and temperature) that characterises supercritical fluids. In the last few years, the research activity in chemistry in gas-expanded solvents has increased significantly. Akien and Poliakoff [24] have recently published a critical review of this research with more than 300 literature references, even after excluding CO_2-polymer and CO_2-ionic liquid media from their publication.

A good proportion of the reactions studied involve gaseous reactants, with a large predominance of hydrogenations. In these cases, the reaction medium is multiphasic (at least biphasic, but triphasic in heterogeneous catalytic systems, where the catalyst is a solid). Phase equilibrium plays here an important role in determining reaction kinetics [25-26].

PARTICLE FORMATION

The first application of gas-expanded solvents was the gas anti-solvent (GAS) recrystallisation, proposed by Gallagher et al [27]. It relies on the decrease of the solvent power of the liquid due to the volume expansion in order to induce precipitation of the solute from the liquid solvent.

The GAS family of techniques is one of the three major groups of methods that use high pressure carbon dioxide for particle formation. The other two are RESS – rapid expansion of supercritical solutions – and PGSS – particles from gas saturated solutions.

Particle formation in these methods is based on the rapid attainment of high supersaturations when fast volume variations occur, and therefore solubilities decrease drastically and very rapidly. These can be induced either by rapid incorporation of high pressure CO_2, as in anti-solvent methods, or rapid decompression of a supercritical solution as in RESS, or of a gas-saturated liquid solution, as in PGSS.

These techniques have raised a lot of interest in the pharmaceutical industry for the formulation of drugs, as they can generate particles of very small size [28-29]. Especially in the case of drug powders for inhalation, where the drug penetrates the blood stream through the lungs, the pharmaceutical industry needed to develop particle engineering and formulation methods that could consistently offer tight control of particle size, morphology, and chemical stability.

In 2000-2001, this interest was translated into acquisitions of companies that had pioneered developments in supercritical fluids, namely Separex, Phasex and Bradford Particle Design. The acquisition of the latter by Inhale Therapeutics was reported to have involved an exchange of shares worth US $200 million. A partnership with Pfizer for the development of inhalable insulin for diabetics raised expectations of a large impact commercial success for this application of supercritical fluids.

Unfortunately this success did not materialise. The FDA approved the first inhaled version of insulin from Pfizer and Sanofi-Aventis in January 2006, and it went into the market in September 2006. A year later, however, Pfizer announced that it would be discontinuing its production, as the drug had failed to gain the acceptance of patients and their doctors.

Notwithstanding, this area of supercritical fluids continues to attract many researchers, and it has been one of the most active in the entire field during the last few years. And although much of the excitement was centred on drug formulation and delivery, varied applications of particle engineering were proposed, including, for instance, coating of materials, and encapsulation of food products [30-31].

SUPERCRITICAL FLUIDS AND MATERIALS

Interaction with and transformation of materials has developed into one of the most studied areas of supercritical fluids. Drug formulation, encapsulation of food products, impregnation of wood, formation of inorganic nanoparticles were some of the examples given above.

One of the most studied fields of application is polymer processing. As already noted, in some favourable cases, supercritical carbon dioxide may be used as solvent for polymer formation. But the applications proposed go much further than synthesis. Polymer- supercritical fluid interactions vary tremendously [32]. They are obviously highly dependent on the chemical nature of the polymer. For many classes of polymers, supercritical carbon dioxide can be used for phase separation, swelling, and viscosity reduction, [33], and foam formation [34].

New applications for biomaterials and bioengineering have been proposed. One interesting area subject to recent attention is the use of supercritical carbon dioxide and natural or synthetic biodegradable polymers to prepare scaffolds for human tissue growth [35-36].

THE FUTURE

Supercritical carbon dioxide and water are extremely attractive solvents in a world where finding solutions for the problem of sustainability is becoming an ever more urgent matter. As a result of 30 years of intensive research, a host of applications has gone commercial, but many others are waiting to be adopted. Often the problems are not technical, but the fact that competing processes are easier and cheaper to apply, although totally unsustainable. In the commemorative issue of the 20th anniversary of the Journal of Supercritical fluids, the potential contributions of technological platforms based on near-critical and supercritical water and carbon dioxide to a more sustainable society have been presented [37-38]. Resistance to change will, as always, be hard to overcome, but it is expectable that many aspects of these proposed platforms will become a reality in the near future.

REFERENCES

[1]   Schneider, G.M. ; Wilke, G. ; Stahl, E. *Extraction with supercritical gases.* Verlag Chemie, Weinheim, *1980*
[2]   McHugh, M.A.; Krukonis V.J. *Supercritical Fluid Extraction, Principles and Practice*; Butterworth-Heinemann, Boston, 1st ed. *1986*, 2nd ed. *1994*
[3]   Stahl, E.; Quirin, K.-W.; Gerard D. *Dense Gases for Extraction and Refining*; Springer-Verlag, Berlin, *1988* – translation of the German version. *J. Supercritical Fluids*, **2009**, 47, 333-636
[4]   Span, R. ; Wagner, W. *J. Phys. Chem. Ref. Data*, **1996**, 25, 1509
[5]   Weingartner, H.; Franck E. U. *Angew. Chem. Int. Ed.*, **2005**, 44, 2672

[6] DeSimone, J.M.; Guan, Z.; Elsbernd, C.S. *Science*, **1992**, 257, 945

[7] Brunner, G. *Gas Extraction*; Steinkopff Verlag, Darmstadt, *1994*

[8] Lack. E. Industrial Cleaning of Cork with Supercritical CO₂. In: Proceedings of the 3rd International Meeting on High Pressure Chemical Engineering; 2006; Erlangen, Germany, pp.1-6

[9] Beckman, E. J. *J. Supercritical Fluids* , **2004**, 28, 121

[10] Iversen, S.B.; Larsen, T.; Henriksen, O.; Felsvang, K. The World's first commercial supercritical wood treatment plant. In: Proceedings of the

[11] Jessop, P. G.; Ikariya, T.; Noyori, R. *Chem. Rev.* **1999**, 99, 475

[12] Jessop, P. G.; Leitner, W.; Eds. *Chemical Synthesis Using Supercritical Fluids*; Wiley VCH: Weinheim, *1999*

[13] Hitzler, M. G.; Smail, F. R. ; Ross, S. K.; Poliakoff, M. *Org.Proc. Res. Dev.* , **1998**, 2, 137

[14] Licence, P.; Ke, J.; Sokolova, M.; Ross, S. K.; Poliakoff, M. *Green Chem.*, **2003**, 5, 99

[15] Du, L.; Kelly, J. Y.; Roberts, G. W. ; DeSimone. J. M. *J. Supercritical Fluids*, **2009**, 47, 447

[16] Brunner, G. *J Supercritical Fluids*, **2009**, 47, 373

[17] Brunner, G. *J Supercritical Fluids*, **2009**, 47, 382

[18] Kruse, A. *J. Supercritical Fluids*, **2009**, 47, 391

[19] Savage, P.E. *J Supercritical Fluids*, **2009**, 47, 407

[20] Augustine, C.; Tester, J.W. *J Supercritical Fluids*, **2009**, 47, 415

[21] Cansell, F.; Aymonier, C. *J. Supercritical Fluids*, **2009**,47, 508

[22] Erkey, C. *J. Supercritical Fluids*, **2009**, 47, 517

[23] Akien, G. R.; Poliakoff, M. *Green Chem.*, **2009**, 11, 1083

[24] Nunes da Ponte, M. *J. Supercritical Fluids*, **2009**, 47, 344

[25] Arai, M. ; Fujita, S.-I. ; Shirai, M. *J. Supercritical Fluids*, **2009**, 47, 351.

[26] Gallagher, P.M.; Coffey, M.P.; Krukonis, V.J.; Klasutis, N. *Gas Antisolvent Recrystallization – New Process to recrystallize Compounds insoluble in Supercritical fluids*. In:ACS Symposium Series 406, American Chemical Society 1989, pp. 334-354.

[27] Türk, M. *J. Supercritical Fluids*, **2009**, 47, 537.

[28] Reverchon, E.; Adami, R.; Cardea, S.; Della Porta, G. *J. Supercritical Fluids*, **2009**, 47,484.

[29] Cocero, M.J.; Martín, A.; Mattea, F.; Varona, S. *J. Supercritical Fluids*, **2009**, 47, 546.

[30] Weidner, E. *J. Supercritical Fluids*, **2009**, 47, 556.

[31] Kikic, I. *J. Supercritical Fluids*, **2009**, 47, 458.

[32] Kiran, E. *J. Supercritical Fluids*, **2009**, 47, 466.

[33] Tomasko, D.L.; Burley, A.; Feng, L.; Yeh, S.-K.; Miyazono, K.; Nirmal-Kumar, S.; Kusaka, I.; Koelling, K. *J. Supercritical Fluids*, **2009**, 47, 493.

[34] Temtem, M.; Silva, L. M. C.; Andrade, P. Z.; da Silva, C. L.; Cabral, J. M. S.; Abecasis, M. M.; Aguiar-Ricardo, A. *J. Supercritical Fluids*, **2009**, 48, 269.

[35] Davies, O. R.; Lewis, A. L.; Whitaker, M. J.; Tai, H.; Shakesheff, K. M.; Howdle, S. M. Adv.Drug Del. Rev. 2008, 60, 373.

[36] King, J. W.; Srinivas, K. *J. Supercritical Fluids*, **2009**, 47, 598.

[37] Arai, K.; Smith Jr., R. L.; Aida, T. M. *J. Supercritical Fluids*, **2009**, 47, 628.

CHAPTER 2

Applications of Supercritical Expansion Processes for Particle Formation

Ana Rita C. Duarte[1,2]*

[1]*3B's Research Group-Biomaterials, Biodegradables and Biomimetics, Dept. of Polymer Engineering, University of Minho, Headquarters of the European Institute of Excellence on Tissue Engineering and Regenerative Medicine, AvePark, Zona Industrial da Gandra, S. Cláudio do Barco, 4806-909 Caldas das Taipas, Guimarães, Portugal, http://www.3bs.uminho.pt and [2]IBB – Institute for Biotechnology and Bioengineering, PT Associated Laboratory (Laboratório Associado), Portugal, www.ibb.pt; Email: aduarte@dep.uminho.pt*

Abstract: Pharmaceutical sciences are experiencing a revolution as regards the existing technologies and the development of entirely new ones. Engineering drug itself has emerged as a new strategy for drug delivery and supercritical fluid technology offers exciting opportunities in this field. The application of supercritical fluids to the processing of pharmaceuticals has already proven its feasibility and also its applicability in the area of polymer processing as well as in the preparation of controlled release systems. It is of particular interest the key role that materials have in the development of these new drug delivery systems, from polymers, to ceramics or even metals. When a pharmaceutical agent is encapsulated within, or attached to, a polymer or lipid, drug safety and efficacy can be greatly improved and new therapies are possible. This has been the driving force for active study of the design of these materials, intelligent delivery systems and approaches for delivery through different administration routes. A review of the state of the art indicates that, in the past two decades, a lot of effort has been put in the development of new particle formation processes. The precipitation of solids with supercritical fluids has attracted many researchers as it enables the production of very small size particles with a narrow size distribution using mild and inert conditions. In this chapter a review of the supercritical expansion processed applied to pharmaceutical purposes is presented.

INTRODUCTION

The importance of biocompatible and biodegradable polymers is continuously increasing in pharmaceutical applications, namely to prepare new controlled drug delivery systems.[1,2] For such systems size and morphology of the polymer matrix assume an extremely important role in the drug release and pharmacokinetics.

Traditionally micronization is carried out at an industrial scale by recrystallization from solution either by spray crystallization or by salting out. [3]

Spray drying has been used by the pharmaceutical industry since the early 40's. It has proven to be a successful technique also for the preparation of microcapsules. This technique is also quite fast and allows the use of mild conditions that prevent the degradation of the product. The production of powders with broad size distributions seems to be the major drawback of this technique.[4]

In the case of the salting out a second liquid solvent is added to the solution with the compound of interest. The anti-solvent is miscible with the primary solvent but it is not miscible with the solute; therefore, as long as the two solvents mix together, the solute precipitates. The drawback of this process is the difficulty in controlling particle size and particle size distribution of precipitates and the elimination of the organic solvent.

In products for medical and pharmaceutical applications, the presence of residual organic solvents is rigorously controlled by international safety regulations. Thus, it is necessary to warrant the complete removal and absence of these substances, without exposing drugs to high temperatures, which may degrade them.[5]

In this sense, supercritical fluids, and particularly supercritical carbon dioxide, are very attractive solvents. Production of micro or nanoparticles using supercritical fluid technology is very attractive since it provides an alternative solution to the various problems encountered in traditional techniques.[6-8] The possibility of producing very small particles with a narrow size distribution using mild and inert conditions represents a major improvement over the conventional processes.[9]

Supercritical carbon dioxide has important advantages when compared to most traditional solvents: is non-toxic, non-flammable and not expensive. Other very important environmental advantage is that the elimination of solvents and the recovery of final products are easier (no residue is left and a dry solid product is easily obtained, just by manipulating pressure), leading to processes with less energy consumption. Carbon dioxide can be recovered and reused, and, therefore, does not contribute to the greenhouse effect. Because of all these advantages, supercritical processes are often referred and classified as "green" and "environmental friendly" processes.

Concerning the processing of pharmaceutical compounds and the preparation of controlled release systems a number of applications and some examples of systems that have been studied are listed in Table **1**:

Table 1: Different applications and examples of the use of supercritical fluid technology for the preparation of controlled release systems

	REFERENCES
Micronization	3,10,11,12
Nanoparticles	13,14
Encapsulation/ Particle coating	15,16, 17
Crystal modification	18,19
Solid dispersions	20,21,22
Dissolution enhancement	23,24,25
Amorphous conversion	26,27
Impregnation	28,29,30
Liposomes	31
Polymerization	32, 33

Intensive world-wide research related with the application of high-pressure and supercritical fluids to particle formation, encapsulation and impregnation of polymeric matrixes has proven the efficiency of supercritical fluid technology to generate improved delivery systems. The growing interest in controlled drug release systems coupled with the strict regulatory legislation are the driver forces for the development of new processes in the pharmaceutical industry. Particularly important issues for this industry are to achieve a clean and environmentally friendly, single-step operation for the production of these systems. Supercritical fluids provide an attractive platform technology to meet the demands of the industry. Nevertheless, any advantage has to be weighted against the cost and inconvenience of the higher pressures needed.

Supercritical fluids comprise several processes, leading to very different particles in terms of size, shape, and morphology. This offers various possibilities to prepare various forms or formulations of the drug: dry inhalable powder, nanoparticle suspension, microspheres or microcapsules of drug embedded in a carrier, drug impregnated excipient or matrix, etc.

Regarding particle formation, different processes are available, [1,34] based on the precipitation from supercritical solutions and precipitation using the supercritical fluid as non-solvent.

When the particles are formed from a compound quite soluble in the supercritical fluid the technique used is RESS. As many pharmaceuticals are almost insoluble in supercritical carbon dioxide, the supercritical anti-solvent process (referred as SAS, ASES, PCA, or SEDS in literature), which uses the anti-solvent effect of supercritical CO_2 to precipitate the substrate(s) initially dissolved in a liquid solvent, is generally considered the most attractive for particle formation and design of improved controlled delivery systems.

This chapter focuses mainly on Supercritical Expansion Processes.

RAPID EXPANSION FROM SUPERCRITICAL SOLUTIONS – SEMI-CONTINUOUS PROCESS

RESS consists in solvating the product in the supercritical fluid and rapidly depressurizing this solution through an adequate nozzle, causing an extremely rapid nucleation of the product into a highly dispersed material. A schematic representation of the process is presented in (Fig. **1**).

The main advantages of the RESS process, include:

- Process of very fine particles
- Controllable particle size
- Solvent free
- Theoretical background rather well understood

The disadvantages of the RESS process are:

- High ratios gas/solute as the solubility of the compounds is usually low in the SCF
- Use of a co-solvent to enhance the solute solubility can result in residual solvent in the final product
- High-pressures and sometimes high temperatures needed for the process
- Large volumes of pressurize equipment required
- Difficult scale-up

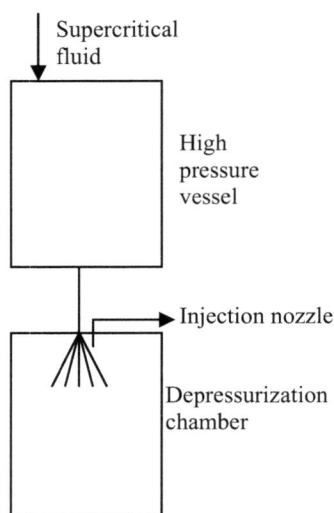

Figure 1: Schematic representation of the semi-continuos RESS process

This concept has been tested for a wide variety of materials including polymers, dyes, pharmaceuticals and inorganic substances. In this survey the main interest are the pharmaceutical and polymer processing applications. Some compounds which have been successfully precipitated from the semi-continuous RESS process are reported in Table **2**:

Table 2: Polymers and pharmaceuticals processed by RESS process.

COMPOUND	REFERENCE
Poly(L-lactic acid)	35,36
Polypropylene	37,38
Benzoic acid	39
Naphthalene	40
Salycilic acid	41,42
Theophylline	43
Naproxen	17
Ibuprofen	44,45
Nifepidine	46
Poly(L-lactic acid) + naproxen	47
Poly(L-lactic acid) + lovastatin	48

In this case, the process works semi-continuously as the depressurization of the vessel occurs through a nozzle, into a lower pressure vessel.

Although this process has been applied to a large range of solutes these are only carried out at bench scale rather than at a semi-pilot or industrial scale. The poor solubility of most compounds in a supercritical fluid is the major limitation of the process which does not assure its economical feasibility.

For this reason, some modifications have been introduced in the past few years to the original supercritical expansion process. Namely the batch processing and the coupling of RESS with fluidized bed, directing the technique to interesting coating applications.

RAPID EXPANSION FROM SUPERCRITICAL SOLUTIONS – BATCH PROCESS

The batch process of the RESS technique is characterized by the precipitation of micro/nano-particles from the supercritical solution by slow depressurization of the high pressure vessel, without the need of a nozzle or any other vessel. (Fig. **2**) represents a schematic illustration of the process:

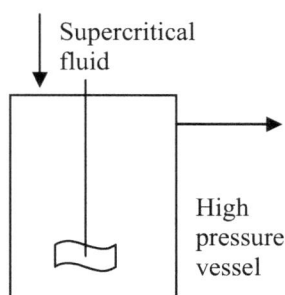

Figure 2: Schematic representation of the batch mode RESS process

This process presents great advantages for the preparation of composite particulate or inclusion systems in which one of the compounds is not soluble in the supercritical phase.

The coating of the active compound is achieved when the carrier (either polymer or lipid) is soluble in the fluid phase and it precipitates upon depressurization of the system over the compound of interest.

Inclusion complexes, such as cyclodextrin/drug complexes can be formed using the same basic principle. In this case, the pharmaceutical agent is dissolved in the supercritical fluid and is transferred to the cyclodextrin cavities, where it will precipitate after the system is depressurized.

Table 3: presents some of the systems reported in the literature prepared by this process.

ACTIVE COMPOUND + CARRIER	REFERENCES
Bovine Serum Albumin + Gelucire Bovine Serum Albumin + Dynasan	16
Piroxicam + β-CD	49
Itraconazole + β-CD	50
Ibuprofen + MBCD	51
Naproxen + β-CD	52

Table 3: Materials processed by batch mode RESS materials

RAPID EXPANSION COUPLED WITH FLUIDIZED BED

The coupling of RESS process with fluidized bed might see interesting applications for coating purposes. This technology has only been explored in the past couple of years and therefore few systems were studied so far. Basically, the coating material is sprayed through a nozzle either from the top or the bottom of a fluidized bed reactor in which the compound to be coated is loaded. The coating process in a fluidized bed can be carried out either in batch mode or continuously. Top spray may lead to the precipitation of granulates whereas bottom spray is advantageous for particle coating. The changed solubility induced by the pressure differences is the driving force for the nucleation. Small particles are formed and adhere to the solid coating the particles. This technique is based on the RESS process, namely on the solubility of a coating agent on the supercritical fluid which is then expanded through an injection nozzle. In this case the depressurization occurs into a fluidized bed reactor, instead of a depressurization chamber. The few studies reported in literature include the coating of model compounds with paraffin, which is known to be soluble in supercritical carbon dioxide. [53-55]

OTHER SUPERCRITICAL EXPANSION PROCESSES

RESOLV- Rapid Expansion of Supercritical carbon dioxide Solutions into a Liquid Solvent

The RESOLV process has the same principle than the semi-continuous RESS process, however in this case the particles are precipitated into an aqueous solution containing a stabilizing agent. Water soluble polymers may be used as stabilizing agents. Different materials have been processed using this technique. Pharmaceuticals, such as paclitaxel [56] and ibuprofen [57] were processed by this technique using different stabilizing agents, such as dodecyl sulfate, poly(N-vinyl-2-pyrrolidone), poly(vinyl alcohol) or poly(ethylene glycol). Fluorinated polymers, due to their solubility in supercritical carbon dioxide have also been precipitated by RESOLV. [58]

DELOS – Depressurization of an Expanded Liquid Organic

The DELOS precipitation technique is a one-step process, which uses a compressed fluid for the production of micro/nano size particles (Fig. 3). The driving force of this process is the fast, large constant temperature decrease experienced by an organic solution in which the compressed fluid is solubilized as it is depressurized to atmospheric pressure.

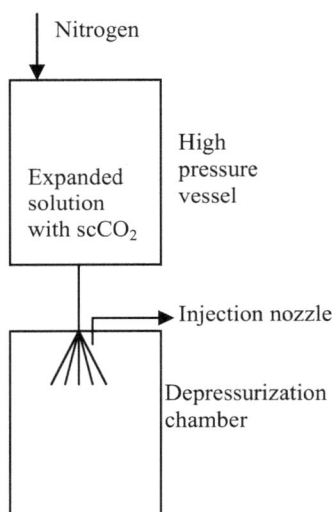

Figure 3: Schematic representation of the DELOS process

The organic solution is in this case expanded by the presence of a supercritical fluid and the depressurization into the lower chamber is carried out at a constant pressure by the introduction of nitrogen in the high-pressure vessel. Nitrogen is the gas chosen as it is inert and will not infer on the composition of the system. In comparison with the other supercritical fluid precipitation techniques in this process the fluid phase acts as co-solvent over the initial organic solution. The DELOS process presents the possibility of the production of fine powders when full miscibility of the ternary system solute + organic solvent + fluid is assured.

Some of the systems prepared using this technique include, the precipitation of 1,4-bis-(n-butylamino)-9,10-anthraquinone [59], ibuprofen and naproxen [69] from acetone + CO_2 solutions.

CAN-BD – Carbon dioxide Assisted Nebulization with Bubble Dryer

The principle underlying the CAN-BD consists on the improvement of the atomization process by the intercalation of liquid droplets and carbon dioxide bubbles in a mixing chamber. [61-63] In this process an aqueous solution and carbon dioxide are mixed in a low-volume tee, before depressurization, forming a spray of aerosols (Fig. **4**). The result is a two-step atomization in which the liquid droplets are broken into smaller ones by the sudden diffusion of CO_2 out of the droplets.

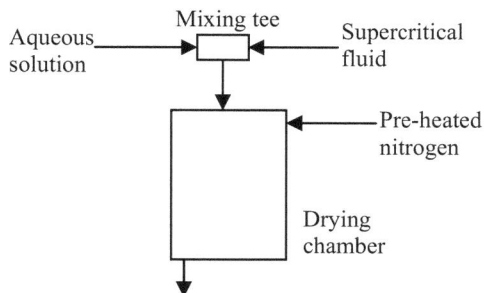

Figure 4: Schematic representation of the CAN-BD process

Thermolabile substances such as active proteins, vaccines and pharmaceuticals have been successfully processed using this technique. [64-65]

PGSS – Particles from Gas Saturated solutions

In the PGSS process, the compound(s) are melted in presence of a compressed gas. The gas dissolved in the liquid phase is then pulverized towards a low-pressure vessel, leading to precipitation of solid particles of compound(s). When a suspension of fine particles of an ingredient dispersed in a liquid excipient is processed, composite microcapsules are generated. (Fig. **5**) illustrates schematically the typical PGSS apparatus:

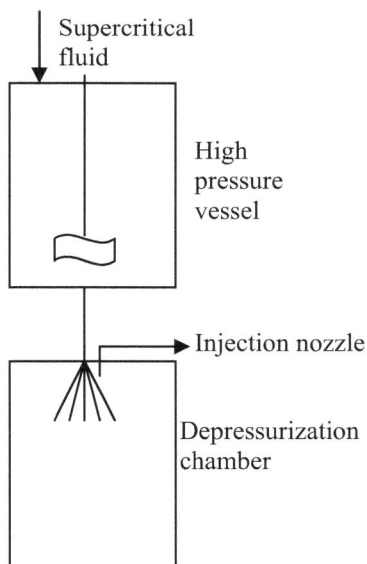

Figure 5: Schematic representation of the PGSS process

The main advantages of this process include the absence of organic solvents, the easy scalability of the process, high production capacity, low pressure of operation and low supercritical consumption. The major drawback is related to the limited applications in the pharmaceutical field.

The application of the PGSS process has been investigated for an extended group of materials, such as: [66]

- polymers (polyethyleneglycols, polyetherurethanes, polymethylmethacrylate),
- waxes and resins,
- natural products (extracts from spices, phospholipids) and
- fat derivatives (partial glycerides, fatty alcohols, fatty acids)

CONCLUSIONS

The choice of the most appropriate process for particle formation depends not only on the solubility of both the active compound and the matrix in the SCF, but also on the solubility of the SCF in the matrixes

The main drawback to the application of SCF technology at the industrial scale is the lack of fundamental studies describing the phase behaviour of the multicomponent systems involved in the processes. The practical implementation of the SCF processes requires full predictability of the product characteristics. Therefore, understanding the influence of the relevant process parameters on the size and shape of the particles formed is a very important key. Being aware of this major weakness, some efforts have been made to describe the phase behaviour, the thermodynamics and hydrodynamics of the processes and some reports on the mechanistic understanding of the SCF processes for particle formation have been published in the past few years. [67-74] The accurate knowledge of mass transfer and nucleation processes will form the basis for efficient scale-up. The commercial viability of a technology depends not only on the main advantages of the technology but also on possibility to scale-up the process. The different SCF formulation processes comprise three main steps for which scale-up is difficult: particle generation, particle collection and fluid purification and recycling. Furthermore, high-pressure operations, namely the use of supercritical fluid technology requires sophisticated control systems for precision and safety, therefore the cost of operation and instrumentation can be quite significative. The progresses made regarding the knowledge of the physical phenomena involved in particle formation coupled to engineering studies will facilitate the development of industrial scale plants and nowadays, already few companies have acquired some know-how in process scale-up, in compliance with GMP (Good Manufacturing Practices) and sterility to produce particles for controlled drug delivery.

REFERENCES

[1]   Yeo, S.-D., Kiran, E., *J. Supercrit. Fluids*, **2005**, 34(3), 287-308
[2]   Shariati, A., Peters, C. J., *Curr. Op. Solid State and Mater. Sci.*, **2003**, 7, 371-383
[3]   Reverchon, E., Porta, G. D., De Rosa, I., Subra, P., Letourneur, D., *J. Supercrit. Fluids*, **2000**, 18 (3), 239-245
[4]   Fu, Y.-J., *et al*, *J. Microencapsulation*, **2001**, 18(6), 733 – 747
[5]   CPMP/ICH/283/95, ICH guideline Q3C, Impurities Residual solvents, **1997**
[6]   Jung, J., Perrut, M., *J. Supercrit. Fluids*, **2001**, 20, 179 – 219
[7]   Fages, J., *et al.*, *Powder Technology*, **2004**, 141, 219-226
[8]   Reverchon, E., Adami, R., *J. Supercrit. Fluids*, **2006**, 37(1), 1-22
[9]   Perrut, M., Clavier, J.-J., *Ind. Eng. Chem. Res.*, **2003**, 42, 6375-6383
[10]   Reverchon, E., Della Porta, G., *J. Supercrit. Fluids*, **2003**, 26(3), 243-252
[11]   Chattopadhyay, P., Gupta, R. B., *Ind. Eng. Chem. Res.*, **2002**, 41(24), 6049-6058
[12]   Kerč, J., Srčič, S., Knez, Ž., Senčar-Božič, P., *Int. J. Pharm.*, **1999**, 182(1), 33-39
[13]   Pathak, P., Meziani, M. J., Desai, T., Sun, Y.-P., *J. Supercrit. Fluids*, 2006, 37 (3), 279-286
[14]   Elvassore, N., Bertucco, A., Calceti, P., *J. Pharm. Sci.*, **2001**, 90, 1628-1636
[15]   Kröber., H., Teipel, U., *Chem. Eng. Proc.*, **2005**, 44, 215–219
[16]   Ribeiro Dos Santos, I., Richard, J., Pech, B., Thies, C., Benoit, J. P., *Int. J. Pharm.*, **2002**, 242(1-2), 69-78
[17]   Kim, J.-H., Paxton, T. E., Tomasko, D. L., *Biotechnol. Prog.*, **1996**, 12(5), 650-661
[18]   Tong, H. H. Y., Shekunov, B. Y., York, P., Chow, A. H. L. , *Pharm. Res.*, **2001**, 18, 852-858
[19]   Gosselin, P. M., Thilbert, R., Preda, M., McMulen, J. N., *Int. J. Pharm.*, **2003**, 252, 225-233
[20]   Juppo, A. M., Boissier, C., Khoo, C., *Int. J. Pharm.*, **2003**, 250(2), 385-401
[21]   Sethia, S., Squillante, E., *Int. J. Pharm.*, **2004**, 272(1-2), 1-10
[22]   Rodier, E., Lochard, H., Sauceau, M., Letourneau, J.-J., Freiss, B., Fages, J., *Eur. J. Pharm. Sci.*, **2005**, 26(2), 184-193
[23]   Nam, K. W., Lee, S. Hawang, S.J., Woo, J.S., Proceedings of the C.R.S. 29th Annual Meeting, **2002**
[24]   Charoenchaitrakool, M., Dehghani, F., Foster, N. R., Chan, H. K., Proceedings of the Fifth International Symposium on Supercritical Fluids, **2000**
[25]   Moneghini, M., Kikic, I., Voinovich, D., Perissutti, B., Filipović-Grĉić, J., *Int. J. Pharm.*, **2001**, 222, 129-138
[26]   Bettini, R., Bnassi, L., Castoro, V., Rossi, A., Zema, L., Gazzaniga, A., Giordano, F., *Eur. J. Pharm. Sci*, **2001**, 13, 281-286
[27]   Tozuka, Y., Kawada, D., Oguchi, T., Yamamoto, K., *Int. J. Pharm.*, **2003**, 263, 45-50
[28]   Kazarian, S. G., Martirosyan, G. G., *Int. J. Pharm.*, **2002**, 232, 81-90
[29]   Elvira, C., Fanovich, A., Fernández, M., Fraile, J., San Román, J., Domingo, C., *J. Controlled Release*, **2004**, 99(2), 231-240
[30]   Duarte, A. R. C., Costa, M. S., Simplício, A. L., Cardoso M. M., Duarte, C.M.M., *Int. J. Pharm.*, **2006**, 308(1-2), 168-174

[31]　Otake, K., Imura, T., Sakai, H., Abe, M., *Langmuir*, **2001**, 17(13), 3898-3901

[32]　Wood, C. D., Cooper, A. I., DeSimone, J. M., *Curr Op Solid State and Mater Sci*, **2004**, 8 (5), 325-331

[33]　Yue, B., Yang, J., Wang, Y., Huang, C.-Y., Dave, R., Pfeffer, R., *Powder Technology*, **2004**, 146(1-2), 32-45

[34]　Foster, N., *et al.*, *Ind. Eng. Chem. Res.*, **2003**, 42, 6476-6493

[35]　Tom, J. W., Debenedetti, P. G., *Biotechnol. Prog.*, **1991**, 7 (5), 403

[36]　Kim, M. Y., Lee, Y. W., Byun, H.-S.; Lim, J. S., *Ind. Eng. Chem. Res.*, **2005**, 45(10), 3388-3392

[37]　Krukonis, V., Presented at the AIChE Annual Meeting, San Francisco, CA, **1984**, Paper 140f.

[38]　Oliveira, J. V., Pinto, J C., Dariva, C., *Fluid Phase Equilibria*, **2005**, 228-229, 381-388

[39]　Domingo, C., Berends, E., Van Rosmalen, G. M., *J. Supercrit. Fluids*, **1997**, 10 (1), 39

[40]　Mohamed, R. S., Halverson, D. S., Debenedetti, P. G., Prud'homme, R. K., *ACS Symp. Ser.*, **1989**, 406, 355.

[41]　Reverchon, E., Donsi, G., Gorgoglione, D., *J. Supercrit. Fluids*, **1993**, 6(4), 241-248

[42]　Huang, Z., Sun, G.-B., Chiew, Y. C., Kawi, S., *Powder Technology*, **2005**, 160(2), 127-134

[43]　Winters, M.A., Frankel, D.Z., Debenedetti, P. G., Carey, J., Devaney, M., Przybycien, T.M., *Biotech. & Bioeng.*, **1999**, 62, 247

[44]　Charoenchaitrakool, M., Dehghani, F., Foster, N. R., Chan,H. K., *Ind. Eng. Chem. Res.*, **2000**, 39 (12), 4794

[45]　Kayrak, D., Akman, U., Hortaçsu, O., *J. Supercrit Fluids*, **2003**, 26(1), 17-31

[46]　Stahl, E., Quirin, K. W., Gerard, D. , Springer-Verlag: New York, **1988**

[47]　Kim, J.-H., Paxton, T. E., Tomasko, D. L., *Biotechnol. Prog.*, **1996**, 12 (5), 650.

[48]　Debenedetti, P. G., Tom, J. W., Kwauk, X., Yeo, S. D., *Fluid Phase Equilib.*, **1993**, 82, 311

[49]　Van Hees, T., Piel, V., Evrard, B., Otte, X., Thunus, L., Delattre, L., *Pharm. Res.*, **1999**, 16, 1864–1870.

[50]　Al-Marzouqi, A.H., Shehatta, I., Jobe, B., Dowaidar, A., *J. Pharm. Sci.* **2006**, 95, 292–304

[51]　Charoenchaitrakool, M., Dehghani, F., Foster, N.R., *Int. J. Pharm.,* **2002**, 239 103–112

[52]　Junco, S., Casimiro, T., Ribeiro, N., da Ponte, M. N., Marques, H.M.C., *J. Inclusion Phenom. Macrocycl. Chem.* **2002**, 44 69–73

[53]　Rodriguez-Rojo, S, Marienfeld, J, Cocero, MJ.., *Chem. Eng. J.*, **2008**, 144(3), 531-539

[54]　Rosenkranz, K, Kasper, MM, Werther J, Brunner, G, *J Supercrit Fluids*, **2008**, 46(3)SI, 351-357

[55]　Schreiber, R, Vogt, C., Werther, J., Brunner G., *J. Supercrit Fluids*, **2002**, 24(2), 137-151

[56]　Pathak, P., Prasad, G.L., Meziani, M.J., Joudeh, A.A., Sun, Y.P., *Langmuir*, **2007**, 23(5), 2674-2679

[57]　Pathak, P., Meziani, M. J., Desai, T., Sun, Y.P., *J. Supercrit. Fluids*, **2006**, 37(3), 279-286

[58]　Sane, A., Thies, M.C., , *J. Phys Chem B*, **2005**, 109(42), 19688-19695

[59]　Ventosa, N., Sala, S., Veciana, J., *J. Supercrit. Fluids*, **2003**, 26 (1), 33-45

[60]　Munto, M., Ventosa, N., Sala, S., Veciana, J., *J. Supercrit. Fluids*, **2008**, 47 (2), 147-153

[61]　Sievers, R.E., Karst, U., USA 5,639,441

[62]　Sievers, R.E., Karst, U., Milewski, P.D., Sellers, S.P., B.A. Miles, B. A., Schaefer, J.D., Stoldt, C. R., Xu, C. Y., *Aerosol Sci. Technol.*, **1999**, 30, 3

[63]　Sievers, R.E., Milewski, P.D., Sellers, S.P., Miles, B.A., Korte, B.J., Kusek, K.D., Clark, G.S., Mioskowski, B., Villa, J.A. *Ind. Eng. Chem. Res.,* **2000,** 39, 4831

[64]　Burger, J.L., Cape, S.P., Braun, C.S., McAdams, D.H., Best, J.A., Bhagwat, P., Pathak, P., Rebits, L.G., Sievers, R.E., *J. Aerosol Med. Pulmonary Drug Deliv,.* **2008**, 21, 25

[65]　Cape, S.P., Villa. J.A., Huang, E.T.S., Yang, T.H., Carpenter, J.F., Sievers, R.E., *Pharm Res*, **2008**, 25 (9), 1967-1990

[66]　Knez, Z., Precipitations of solids with dense gases, Lecture notes from Socrates intensive program on high-pressure chemical enginering processes, Barcelona, **2004**

[67]　Palakodaty, S., York, P., ***Pharm. Res.,*** **1999**, 16(7), 976-985

[68]　Shariati, A., Peters, C.J., *J. Supercrit. Fluids*, **2002**, 23, 195-208

[69]　Mukhopadhyay, M., Dalvi, S.V., *J. Supercrit. Fluids*, **2004**, 30, 333-348

[70]　Martín, A., Cocero, M.J., *J. Supercrit Fluids*, **2004**, 32, 203-219

[71]　Elvassore, N., Flaibani, M., Bertucco, A., Caliceti, P., *Ind. Eng. Chem. Res.*, **2003**, 42(23), 5924-5930

[72]　Elvassore, N., Cozzi, F., Bertucco, A., *Ind. Eng. Chem. Res.*, **2004,** 43(16), 4935-4943

[73]　Lora, M., Bertucco, A., Kikic, I., *Ind. Eng. Chem. Res.*, **2000**, 39(5), 1487-1496

[74]　Kikic, I., Lora, M., Bertucco, A., *Ind. Eng. Chem. Res.*, **1997**, 36(12), 5507-5515

Supercritical Anti-Solvent Micronization: Control of Morphology and Particle Size

Ernesto Reverchon* and Iolanda De Marco

Università degli Studi di Salerno, Dipartimento di Ingegneria Chimica e Alimentare, Via Ponte Don Melillo, 1 - 84084, Fisciano (SA), Italy, Email: ereverchon@unisa.it

Abstract: Supercritical antisolvent precipitation has been used to micronize several kinds of materials. Nanoparticles with mean diameters in the 30-200 nm range and microparticles in the 0.2-20 μm range are the most frequently obtained morphologies. Sometimes, hollow expanded microparticles with diameters between about 10 and 200 μm and crystals having various morphologies have been obtained. In this work, the relation between vapor liquid equilibria and the observed morphologies has been performed; possible formation mechanisms have been proposed. If the material is precipitated from a supercritical gaseous phase, expanded microparticles can be obtained; whereas, if the process is carried out at supercritical conditions, there is a competition between jet break-up and liquid surface tension vanishing characteristic times. If surface tension disappears before the jet break-up, nanoparticles are formed from a gas plume; otherwise, micrometric droplets generate spherical micrometric particles.

INTRODUCTION

Micronization processes based on the use of supercritical carbon dioxide have been extensively tested during the last years as alternatives to the traditional techniques [1-3]. Among the proposed processes, the Supercritical AntiSolvent (SAS) precipitation has been largely used in several research areas: pharmaceuticals, superconductors, coloring matters, explosives, polymers, biopolymers, etc. Several particles morphologies have been recurrently obtained by SAS: nanoparticles with mean diameters in the 30-200 nm range, microparticles in the 0.2-20 μm range, expanded hollow microparticles (balloons) with diameters between about 10 and 200 μm and various crystals morphologies [1-4]. Several SAS operating parameters, like pressure, temperature, concentration in the liquid solution and carbon dioxide molar fraction, together with liquid jet characteristics, can influence particle size (PS) and particle size distribution (PSD) [5-8].

Generally speaking, nanoparticles have been obtained for several compounds at pressures much larger than the mixture critical point (MCP) of the binary system solvent-supercritical antisolvent [9-11]. Microparticles have been generally obtained at near critical conditions and can also show various degrees of cristallinity, though they in the most cases were found to be amorphous [5, 6, 12-14]. Microparticles with hollow or porous interiors have also been produced for compounds belonging to different categories, using different liquid solvents, operating at subcritical gas phase conditions [15-18].

Some authors discussed the precipitation mechanisms and the interactions of mass transfer, atomization and vapor liquid equilibria (VLEs) of the system solvent-antisolvent to obtain a successful SAS precipitation [9, 11, 16, 17, 19, 20]. The morphology of the precipitated powder can be function of the position of the operating point with respect to the MCP of the ternary system. A common hypothesis is that the ternary phase diagram formed by the solute, solvent and antisolvent substantially behaves like the binary system solvent-antisolvent. However, using this hypothesis, some of the observed SAS behaviors cannot be explained [7]. Some attempts have also been made to propose a mathematical modelling of the formation mechanisms of SAS observed particles morphologies. But, very limited sets of data have been generally used or ideal conditions have been postulated, like single stationary droplet analysis [21-23].

Thus, until now a general description of the SAS operating conditions to be used to produce the various kind and size of particles experimentally observed has not been proposed. The scope of this work is to organize the results obtained using SAS and to discuss the mechanisms generating different morphologies and dimensions of precipitates.

Ana Rita C. Duarte & Catarina M. M. Duarte (Eds)

TYPICAL SAS EXPERIMENTAL APPARATUS AND PROCEDURES

A typical semi-continuous SAS apparatus is represented in Fig. **1**. It consists of a high pressure pump used to feed the liquid solution and a diaphragm high-pressure pump, equipped with a cooling system for the pumping head, used to deliver liquid carbon dioxide. A high pressure vessel is used as the precipitation chamber. The liquid mixture is usually sprayed in the precipitator through a thin wall stainless steel nozzle through an inlet port located on the top of the chamber; other injector configurations are also used, as, for example, capillary nozzles. CO_2 is heated to the process temperature before entering the precipitator. A stainless steel frit is generally put at the bottom of the precipitation chamber to collect the solid product, allowing the CO_2–organic solvent solution to pass through. A second vessel located downstream the micrometering valve is used to recover the liquid solvent. A back-pressure valve regulates the pressure in this vessel. At the exit of the second vessel, rotameters and dry test meters are commonly used to measure the CO_2 flow rate and the total quantity of antisolvent delivered.

A common variation of the semicontinuous SAS process is the discontinuous SAS (named GAS) in which the liquid solution is put in the precipitator at the beginning of the experiment and, then, CO_2 is pumped into the vessel up to the final set pressure [24-27]. This process shares various similarities with SAS; but, it never operates at steady state conditions since the pressure continuously varies from 1 bar to the final test pressure. Also the atomization step is missing. Therefore, it is more than probable that the precipitation mechanisms will be different than in SAS [28].

In some cases, pilot plants have been used for the micronization experiments [13, 29, 30]. They are very similar to the laboratory scale ones, but differ from the bench scale ones regarding the injection system, that is generally a tube in tube device. As a rule, the pilot plant operates in closed loop: CO_2 is recycled after the decompression step. Windowed precipitators have also been used to investigate the macroscopic evolution of the SAS process. In this case, the precipitator is equipped with quartz windows that allow the visual observation of the jet break-up and of the precipitation phenomena.

A SAS experiment begins by the delivery of supercritical CO_2 at a constant flow rate to the precipitation chamber until the desired pressure is reached. Then, pure solvent is sent through the nozzle to the chamber with the aim of obtaining steady state composition conditions of the fluid phase during the solute precipitation. The solvent is also delivered to avoid blockage of the injection nozzle due to the precipitation of solute during the start up phase. When steady state conditions have been obtained, the flow of the liquid solvent is stopped and the liquid solution is delivered through the nozzle at a given flow rate. In some cases, the liquid solution is directly sent to the precipitator. Once a given quantity of organic solution is injected and solute has been precipitated, the liquid pump is stopped; however, supercritical CO_2 continues to flow to wash the chamber, eliminating the supercritical solution formed by the liquid solubilized in the supercritical antisolvent. If the final purge with pure CO_2 is not performed, the solvent contained in the fluid phase condenses during the depressurization step and can solubilize or modify the precipitates. At the end of the washing step, CO_2 flow is stopped and the precipitator is depressurized down to atmospheric pressure.

Several organic solvents have been used in SAS experiments; the most used are dimethylsulfoxide (DMSO), N-methylpyrrolidone (NMP), ethanol (EtOH), methanol (MeOH), dichloromethane (DCM), but, also chloroform ($CHCl_3$), acetone (AC), isopropanol (C_3H_7OH), dimethyl formamide (DMF), formic acid (HCOOH), ethyl acetate (EtAc), acetic acid (AA) have been used.

Samples of the processed powders are as a rule observed by scanning electron microscopy. Particle size (PS) and particle size distributions (PSDs) can be measured by an analysis performed on SEM images to measure and count the particles, using a dedicated software or a dynamic laser scattering apparatus.

X-ray diffraction (XRD) and differential scanning calorimetry (DSC) analyses have also been performed to ascertain if changes occurred in the crystal habit and crystallinity of the materials, as a consequence of the SAS processing.

SELECTION OF THE OPERATING PARAMETERS FOR SUCCESSFUL SAS MICRONIZATION

The prerequisites for successful SAS processing are the complete miscibility between the liquid solvent and the antisolvent and the insolubility of the solute in the antisolvent; or, more precisely, in the solution solvent–antisolvent formed in the precipitator. Considering the binary system solvent–antisolvent, at a given temperature, this condition is obtained at pressures larger than the mixture critical point (MCP); it represents, in a pressure-composition plane, the pressure at which only a single supercritical phase can exist. However, it should be also considered that the

Presence of a solute, if it is soluble in the system solvent + antisolvent, can modify the binary system vapor–liquid equilibria (VLEs). As a rule, the MCP of the ternary system moves towards higher pressures than for the corresponding binary one [7, 8, 31]. In SAS experiments performed using windowed precipitator, it has been observed that the ternary system could be at subcritical conditions even when the corresponding liquid–CO_2 binary system is supercritical [6, 29].

However, despite these general considerations, the literature indicates that SAS experiments have been performed in a relatively small range of temperatures (as a rule, 35 to 60 °C), but in a wide range of pressures that comprises also subcritical, liquid and two-phase conditions and spans from about 60 to 250 bar. Varying the operating conditions, different morphologies; i.e., crystals, nanoparticles, microparticles and expanded microparticles, have been obtained.

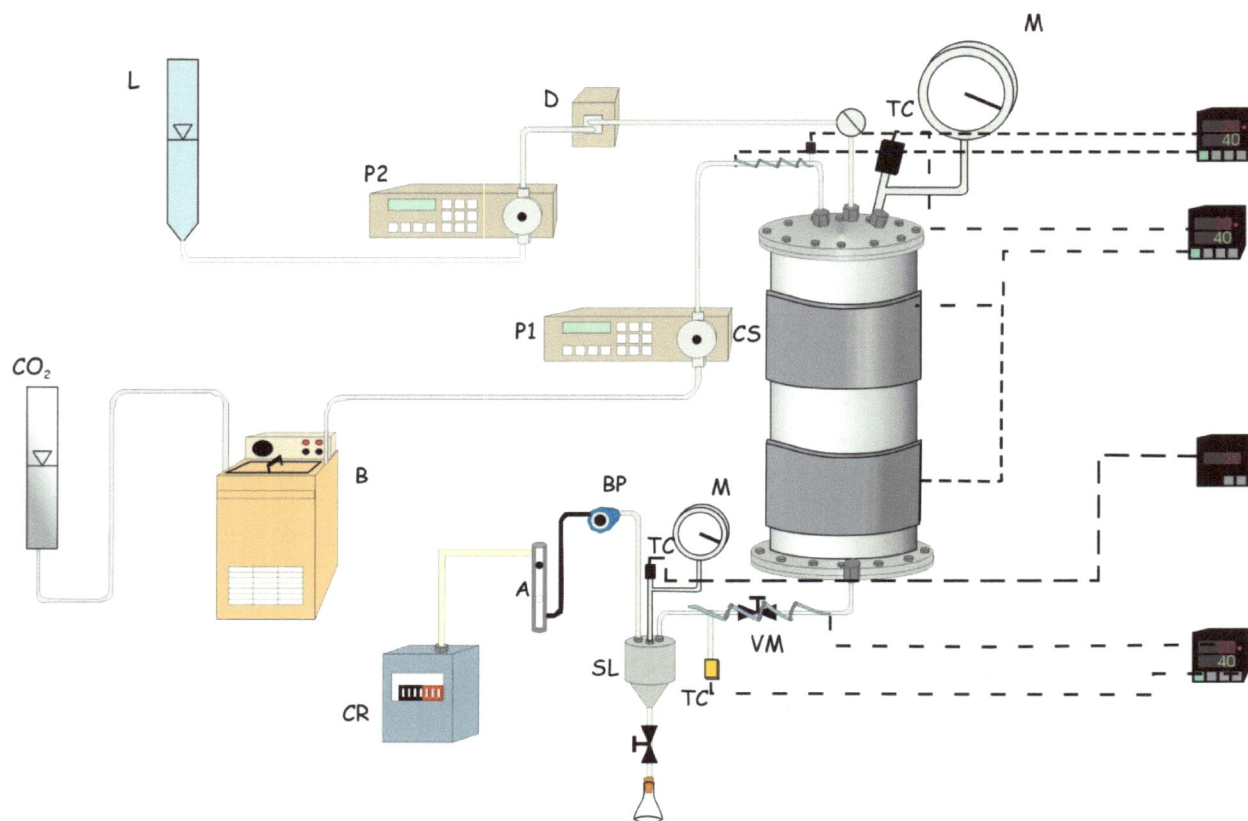

Figure 1: Schematic representation of a SAS apparatus: L, liquid supply; B, refrigerating bath; P1–P2, pumps; D, pressure dampener; CS, precipitation vessel; M, manometer; TC, thermocouple; VM, micrometering valve; SL, liquid separator; BP, back-pressure valve; A, calibrated rotameter; CR, wet test meter.

MORPHOLOGIES

Expanded Microparticles

These particles are perfectly spherical and are characterized by an empty shell morphology. Their diameter can range from some to several tenths of micrometers up to 200 μm.

This morphology has been observed for several compounds, such as yttrium acetate, zinc acetate, samarium acetate, cellulose acetate, dextran, cefonicid, polyvinylalcohol (PVA) and salbutamol [7, 8, 15, 28, 29, 32-34]. In Table **1**, a list of some SAS processed materials has been reported with the indication of the various obtained morphologies; i.e., nanoparticles, microparticles and Expanded MicroParticles (EMP).

Expanded microparticles can show two different surface morphologies: continuous surface or connected nanoparticles surface. Examples of continuous surface are reported in Figs. **2a** and **2b**; no discontinuity of the surface is observed even at microscopic level.

The expanded microparticles with connected nanoparticles surface are exemplified in Figs. **3a** and **3b**. At microscopic level, they show a discontinuous surface formed by interconnected nanoparticulate elements.

Expanded microparticles have been observed only when SAS process has been performed at subcritical gaseous conditions for the binary system solvent – antisolvent.

Microparticles

They are perfectly spherical particles whose diameter can range from about 0.2 to 20 μm. Microparticles have been observed for many kind of compounds as shown in Table **1**; practically all the categories of compounds tested by SAS are represented in this morphology: superconductor precursors, pharmaceuticals, polymers, etc.

Differently from the expanded particles analyzed in the previous chapter, these particles do not show an internal structure (they are not empty) and their surface is continuous even at microscopic level. Examples of microparticles produced by SAS are reported in Figs. **4a** and **4b** and are referred to rifampicin and cefonicid, respectively. Particle size distribution of these particles has been calculated by analysis of SEM images or using dynamic laser scattering (DLS). A typical example of microparticle size distribution is reported in Fig. **5**.

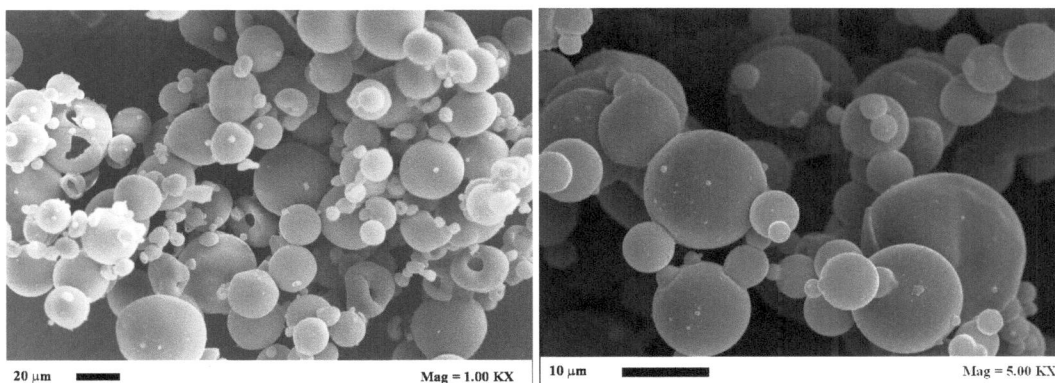

Figure 2: Expanded continuous surface microparticles. a) Dextran precipitated from DMSO at 150 bar, 65 °C and 0.91 % wt; b) PVA precipitated from DMSO at 120 bar, 60 °C and 0.91 % wt.

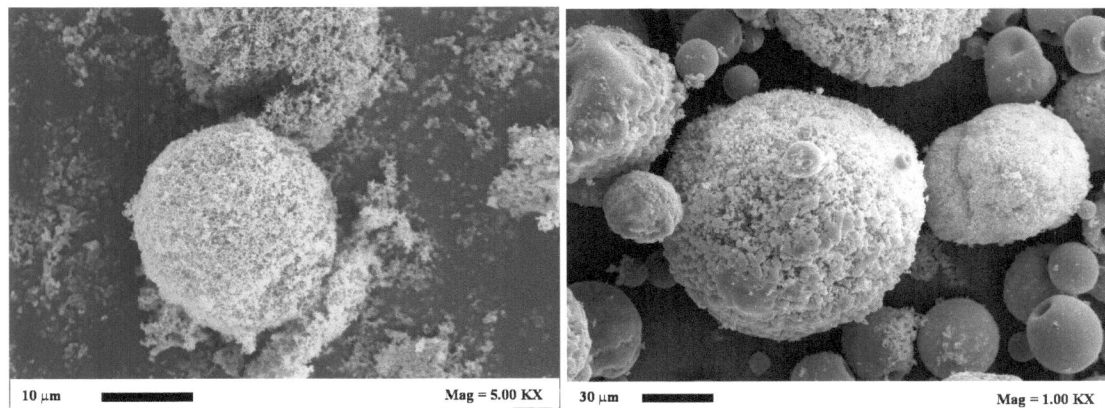

Figure 3: Expanded nanostructured microparticles. a) Cellulose acetate precipitated from acetone at 90 bar, 60 °C and 1.27 % wt; b) Yttrium acetate precipitated from DMSO at 150 bar, 65 °C and 4.55 % wt.

This particle morphology has been prevalently observed when the SAS process has been performed in the relative proximity of the mixture critical point (MCP) in a region of pressure of about 10 to 30 bar higher than the MCP pressure of the specific solvent-antisolvent mixture used.

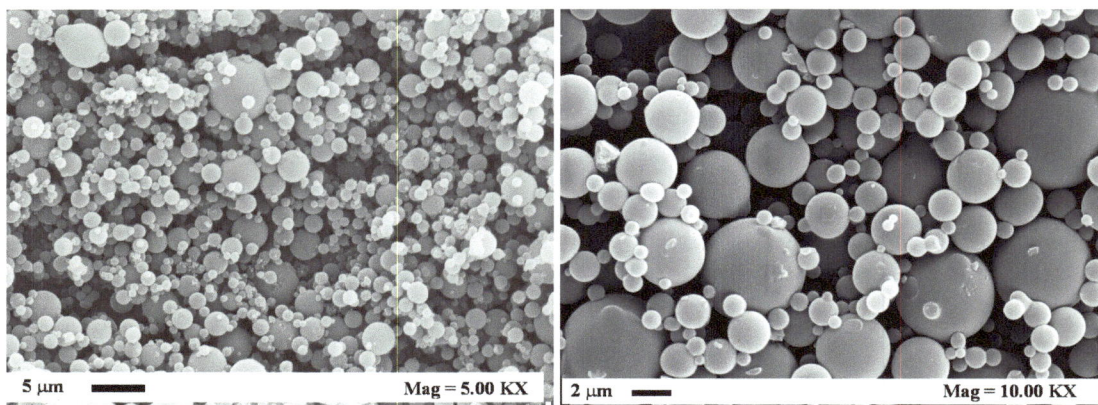

Figure 4: Microparticles. a) Rifampicin precipitated from DMSO at 95 bar, 40 °C and 0.91 % wt; b) Cefonicid precipitated from DMSO at 150 bar, 60 °C and 1.37 % wt.

Nanoparticles

They are irregularly spherical and in some cases are coalescent. In some limited cases the aggregation is due to the formation of solid bridges connecting groups of nanoparticles [9]. In all the other cases, it should be possible to produce single nanoparticles by, for example, ultrasonication. Their mean diameter can range from 30 to about 200 nanometers. An accurate analysis of the influence of the starting concentration of the liquid solution on nanoparticles diameters has been performed elsewhere [9].

Nanoparticles have been observed for many SAS processed compounds as shown in Table **1**. Some examples of SAS produced nanoparticles are shown in Figs. **6a** and **6b**.

Their surface morphology do not present any substructure. It is relevant that, in this case, it does not exist a precise geometry of the particles: they maintain a spherical shape and, when collected in the precipitator vessel, they are not collapsed on the bottom of the vessel, but present a high volume fractal-like geometry that can be destroyed during the powder collection.

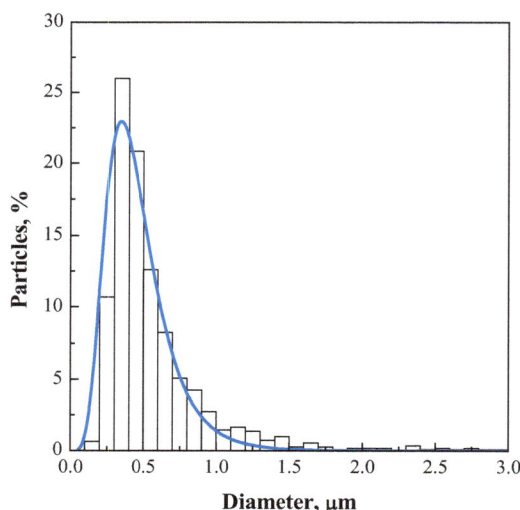

Figure 5: Particle size distribution of □-Cyclodextrin/DMSO particles obtained at 150 bar, 40 °C, 9.1 % wt.

These kind of particles have been produced (see Table **1**) when SAS process has been performed at pressures relatively higher than the MCP pressure (pressures about 30-50 bar or more higher the MCP).

It is worth of note that the pressure ranges typical of microparticles and nanoparticles can partly overlap; this will be one of the fact to be clarified in the following discussion.

Crystals

The formation of crystals ranging from some microns to hundreds of microns has been frequently reported; in most cases, acicular crystals have been observed [67-71]. Working with the same solvent and antisolvent, and at the same operating conditions (for example, 150 bar, 40 °C, x_{CO2}= 0.97), the formation of microparticles [58] or of large crystals [35] has been observed; the only difference being the solute. An example of crystalline particles is reported in Fig. **7**.

MECHANISMS THAT CAN EXPLAIN THE MORPHOLOGIES OBSERVED

As stated in the introduction, the SAS precipitation mechanism is a complex interplay of thermodynamics, mass transfer and fluidodynamic effects. The proper selection of the atomization device and of the process conditions to obtain the jet break-up and the droplets formation is relevant. The jet break-up of the liquid jet at the exit of the injector is driven by the competition among cohesive and disruptive forces. Surface tension and viscosity of the liquid jet are the cohesive forces; whereas, the friction between the liquid jet and the surrounding gas and jet turbulence are the disruptive forces. Different jet break-up regimes are possible and correlations between Weber (or Ohnesorge) and Reynolds numbers and the various break-up regimes are available in the literature [71].

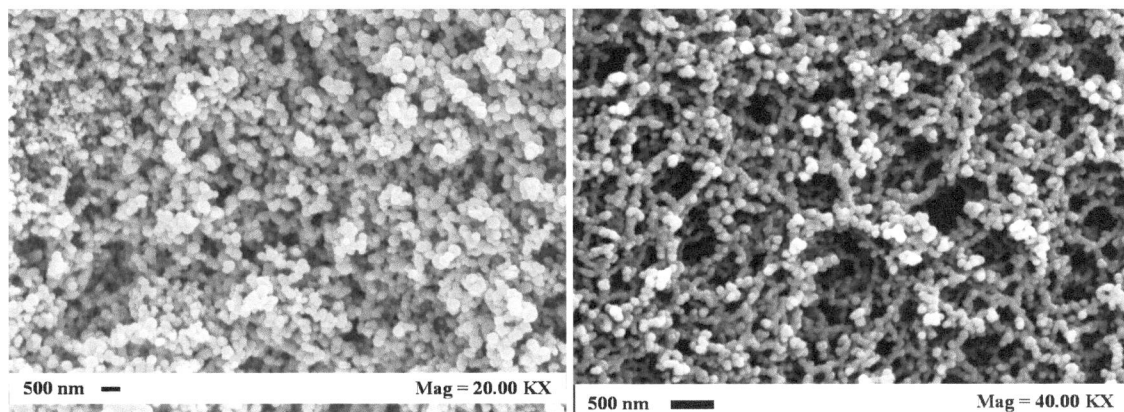

Figure 6: Nanoparticles. a) Europium acetate precipitated from DMSO at 150 bar, 40 °C and 9.1 % wt; b) Rifampicin precipitated from Methanol at 150 bar, 40 °C and 0.91 % wt.

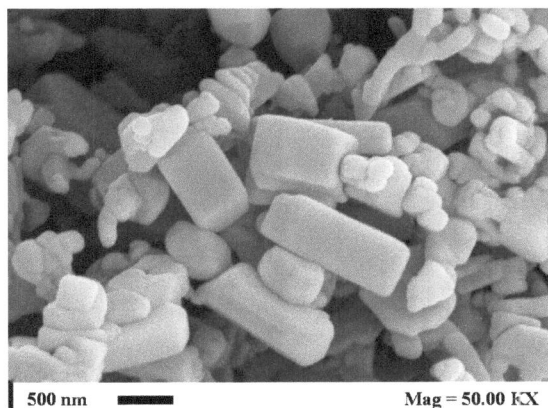

Figure 7: Crystals of Dexamethasone precipitated from acetone at 85 bar, 40 °C and 1.26 % wt.

The phase behavior of the binary system solvent-CO_2 is usually a type-I system in the classification proposed by van Konynenburg and Scott [72]. Its behavior is characteristic of systems formed by a supercritical component (like CO_2) and a medium volatility solvent; an example of such systems is reported in Fig. **8**. The third compound, the solid, can modify the phase behavior of the binary mixture; but, in many cases, it can be considered negligible, when low concentrations of solute are used. However, it is worth to note that this is an over-simplification because several solutes, even at low concentrations, can raise the dew point pressure of the mixture [7, 8, 29].

Table 1: Morphologies obtained with the SAS process.

Solute	Solvent	P, bar	T, °C	C, % wt	morphology	d[μm]	Ref
Pharmaceuticals, proteins and enzymes							
5-fluorouracil	DCM/EtOH 80/20 v/v	120	33	sat.	microparticles	<0.5	[40]
α-Cyclodextrin	DMSO	150	40	0.91-18.2	microparticles	0.2-5	[14, 40]
β-Cyclodextrin	DMSO	150	40	2.73-18.2	microparticles	0.3-4	[14, 41]
Amoxicillin	NMP	150	40	1.94	nanoparticles	0.118	[5, 12, 30]
	NMP	150	35-50	1.94-9.72	microparticles	0.25-0.8	[5, 30]
	DMSO	100-250	40	0.5-2.0	microparticles	0.47-0.86	[41]
	DMSO/EtOH 50/50 v/v	100-250	40	1.0	microparticles	0.35-0.43	[42]
Ampicillin	NMP	150	40	1.95	microparticles	0.26	[42]
	DMSO	150	40	1.36	nanoparticles	0.045	[12]
Astemizole	DMSO	150	40	0.45-0.91	nanoparticles	0.095-0.115	u.r.
Atorvastatin calcium	MeOH	100-120	40-60	6.3-18.9	microparticles	0.26-0.86	[43]
Cefonicid	DMSO	120-150	40	4.54	microparticles	0.3-1.35	[7, 8]
		150	40	8.17	microparticles	18	[7]
		100	50	0.91	Uniform EMP		[8]
		150	60	0.91-2.27	microparticles	1.5-3	[8]
Cefoperazone	DMSO	150	40	0.91-8.17	microparticles	0.25-0.51	[8]
Insulin	DMSO	86.2	25-35	0.45-1.36	microparticles	1.87-2.68	[44]
	DMF	86.2	35	0.53	microparticles	2.48	[45]
Ipratropium bromide	DMF	160-200	40-50	1.06	microparticles	1.86-4.48 irregular and aggregated	[45, 46]
	EtOH/AC 34/66 v/v	200	40-50	1.27-1.91	microparticles	5.04-6.74 irregular and aggregated	[46]
Lysozyme	DMSO	85.8-150	34-50	0.20-1.0	microparticles	1.94-5.28 aggregated	[47, 48]
Nalmefene HCl	EtOH	120-150	60-67	1.9	microparticles	0.9-4.5	[13]
Rifampicin	DMSO	95-100	40	0.91-6.36	microparticles	0.85-1.14	[6]
	DMSO	150	40	0.27-0.91	nanoparticles	0.07-0.115	
	MeOH	150	40	1.27	nanoparticles	0.06	
	EtAc	150	40	0.56	nanoparticles	0.07	
	DCM	150	40	0.38	nanoparticles	0.1	
Salbutamol	DMSO	90	40	0.45	Crystalline EMP		[14, 34]
Soy lecithin	EtOH	80-110	35	5.0-16.5	microparticles	1-45 aggregated	[49]
Sulphatiazole	AC	80	50	1.9	microparticles	1-5	[50]
Terbutaline sulphate	EtOH/DMF (95/5 v/v)	180	40	0.63	nanoparticles	0.2-0.3 irregular and aggregated	[47]
	EtOH/DMF (90/10 v/v)	140	40	0.62	nanoparticles	0.2-0.3 irregular and agglomerated	
	EtOH/DMF (50/50 v/v)	180	40	0.58	nanoparticles	0.3-0.5 irregular and aggregated	
Superconductor precursors							
Europium Acetate	DMSO	150	40	0.91-9.1	nanoparticles	0.06-0.15	[51]
		150	40	9.1-27.25	microparticles	0.24-0.27	
Gadolinium Acetate	DMSO	150	40	0.45-4.36	nanoparticles	0.055-0.15	[52]
		150	40	1.82-31.8	microparticles	0.21-0.4	

Neodymium Acetate	DMSO	150	40	0.45	nanoparticles	0.067	[32]
Samarium Acetate	DMSO	90	40	1.36	Nanostructured EMP		[14]
		150	40	0.18-2.36	nanoparticles	0.047-0.13	[32]
Yttrium Acetate	DMSO	150	40	0.45-3.27	nanoparticles	0.05-0.12	[29, 32]
		70-150	40-50	1.36-13.6	microparticles	0.24-25	[29]
		90	40	1.36	Nanostructured EMP		[29, 32]
		150	43	9.1	microparticles	5	[14]
		120	50-60	1.36	Nanostructured EMP		[29, 32]
		150	65	4.5	Nanostructured EMP		[29]
		120-135	60	4.5	Nanostructured EMP		[14]
		150	65	4.5	Uniform EMP		[14]
		160	70	1.36	Nanostructured EMP		[29]
Catalyst precursors							
Zinc Acetate	DMSO	90	40	1.36	Nanostructured EMP		[33]
		150	40	0.45-6.82	nanoparticles	0.045-0.15	
	NMP	150	40	0.97	nanoparticles	0.055	
Explosives							
Nitrotriazole	DMSO	150	40	1.82	nanoparticles	0.065	u.r.
Polymers							
Cellulose Acetate	Ac	150	40	1.27	nanoparticles	0.125	u.r.
		90	60	1.27	Nanostructured EMP		u.r.
mCOC	Toluene	150	40	0.25-2	nanoparticles	0.041-0.0628	[52]
	o-Xylene	150	40	1	nanoparticles	0.05	
	m-Xylene	150	40	1	nanoparticles	0.0528	
	p-Xylene	150	40	1	nanoparticles	0.0535	
	THF	150	40	1	nanoparticles	0.0425	
Nylon 6/6	HCOOH	88	40	0.6-1.2	microparticles	2.9	[53]
PHB[2]	DCM	90-200	40	1.5	microparticles	2.23-5.77 aggregated	[54]
PHBV[3]	DCM	80-100	35-40	0.96	microparticles	5.8-8.3	[55]
PHBV[3]	CHCl3	100	40	0.96	microparticles	5.3	[56]
Biopolymers							
3bPLG[1]	DCM/TFE[2] 98.7/1.3 w/w	100	34	0.38	microparticles	6	[56]
Dextran 40	DMSO	150	40	0.23-1.36	nanoparticles	0.05-0.125	[57]
		150	65	0.91	Uniform EMP		
HPMA	DMSO	150	40	0.91	nanoparticles	0.085	[58]
HYAFF 11	DMSO	150	40	0.91	nanoparticles	0.095	u.r.
Inulin	DMSO	150	40	2.27	nanoparticles	0.1	[58]
		150	40	4.54	microparticles	0.8-1	u.r.
PLGA 50/50	DCM/TFE[4] 98.7/1.3 w/w	100	34	0.38	microparticles	17 aggregated	[57]
PLLA	DCM	75-350	31-60	0.08-5.0	microparticles	0.5-13.7 irregular	[23, 55, 58-68]
	CHCl3	85.8-101.1	35-40	0.47-1.0	microparticles	1-3.5	[11, 68]
	DCM/DMSO (75/25 w/w)	100	33	0.1	microparticles	1-4 aggregated	[62]
	DCM/DMSO (50/50 w/w)	100-130	32-39	0.1	microparticles	1.5 aggregated	[62]
	DCM/CHCl3 (8/92 v/v)	140	34	0.23	microparticles	12.3 irregular	[69]
PVA	DMSO	120-140	60	0.91-3	Uniform EMP		[14, 28]
		150	40	0.91	nanoparticles	0.060	u.r.

Colouring matters							
Bronze Red	AC	80-120	35-75	0.13	microparticles	3-6	[70]
	EtOH	80-120	35-75	0.13	microparticles	1-8	[71]
Disperse Red 60	DMSO	150	40	0.45-1.36	nanoparticles	0.058-0.102	[31]
	NMP	150	40	0.48-1.45	nanoparticles	0.093-0.112	
	Ac	150	40	1.27	nanoparticles	0.1	
Solvent Blue 35	NMP	150	40	0.48	nanoparticles	0.07	u.r.
	Ac	150	40	0.63	nanoparticles	0.07	u.r.
Solvent yellow 56	NMP	150	40	1.94	nanoparticles	0.07	u.r.
	Ac	150	40	2.53	nanoparticles	0.115	u.r.

[1] 3bPLG is (b-poly-L-lactide-co-D, L-lactide-co-glycolide 62: 5: 12: 5: 25);

[2] PHB is poly(β-hydroxybutyric acid);

[3] PHBV is poly(3-hydroxybutyrate-*co*-3-hydroxyvalerate);

[4] TFE is 2, 2, 2-Trifluoroethanol;

EMP = expanded microparticles; , u.r. = unpublished results

Mass transfer, between the liquid and the gaseous phase, is the process that induces the precipitation of the solute. The mass transfer from gas phase to the liquid phase dominates this process; however, the final morphology of the solids is also conditioned by the kinetics of nucleation and growth that is specific of the solute involved.

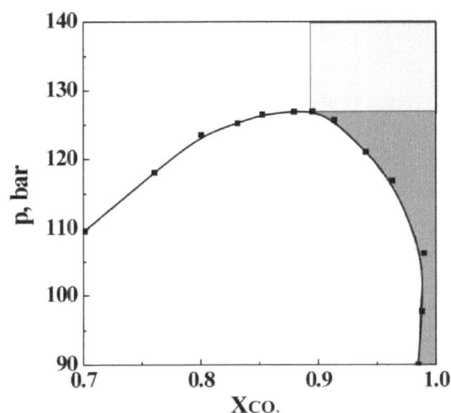

Figure 8: Part of the P–x diagram for the binary system DMSO–CO$_2$ at 55 °C (adapted from [18]).

Expanded Microparticles

Expanded microparticles have been obtained when SAS has been operated at subcritical conditions, as a rule, for values of $x_{CO_2} \geq 0.97$ (see the zone indicated in dark grey in Fig. **8**). When liquid droplets are generated by atomization in a subcritical gas phase, the surface tension of the liquid does not go to zero and its presence forces the droplets to maintain the spherical shape.

Therefore, a possible mechanism for expanded microparticles formation is the following: CO$_2$ diffuses inside the droplet and (in a minor extent) the organic solvent diffuses in the surrounding gas. The droplets are expanded by dissolved CO$_2$ and the presence of the surface tension stabilizes the expanded droplet. The mass transfer of gaseous CO$_2$ inside the liquid also progressively reduces the surface tension, that is, however, strong enough to maintain the shape of the droplet. This behavior is also supported by various studies on liquid expansion produced by SC-CO$_2$, in which a massive expansion of the liquid has been observed.

The numerical analysis performed by Werling and Debenedetti [21] on the behavior of a single toluene droplet into a subcritical CO$_2$ environment also confirms this mechanism. These authors considered the time-dependent conservation equations coupled to an equation of state and calculated mass transfer inside (diffusion) and outside (evaporation) the single droplet. They showed that the droplet largely expands with respect to the initial diameter until the two fluxes at the interface are balanced. The precipitation of solute (not considered in the model of Werling and Debenedetti [21]) produces a solid shell that remains intact after the end of the mixing between solvent and antisolvent. The final result is that the droplet expands like a "balloon" in which a gas is blown, until the precipitation of solute starts. The highest CO_2 concentration is at the droplet surface; therefore, during the expansion process the solute reaches the saturation at the surface and starts to precipitate. We also observed that all the remaining part of solute tends to accumulate on this solid surface, producing hollow shells. There are two possible explanations for this last process. First, the diffusion of CO_2 in the liquid droplet produces also a convective movement of the liquid; therefore, the internal of the droplet behaves as a stirred tank reactor, in which the concentration of the solute is uniform in all the volume except at a boundary layer located near the walls, in which the concentration of the solute is very high, leading to saturation and precipitation of new solid contributes. Second, the liquid solution contained in the droplet is stagnant and a concentration profile of solute is established with the minimum at the center of the droplet and the maximum near the surface. This profile is induced by the diffusion of CO_2 from the surface of the droplet to its center. Also in this case, the solute reaches the saturation near the surface of the droplet and precipitates, producing a progressive thickening of the solid wall. At the end of the process, a hollow micrometric particle with the diameter equal to the final expansion of the droplet is obtained, in which all the solid is accumulated near the surface. This mechanism of "droplet confined liquid expansion" is, thus, able to explain the formation of the expanded micro-particles. This mechanism is also consistent with the production of EMP formed by the simultaneous precipitation of two compounds. Indeed, both compounds are contained in each droplet and their precipitation is confined by the droplet volume and by their accumulation on the droplet surface.

Microparticles

Summarizing the experimental observations at pressure near above supercritical conditions for the binary mixture liquid-CO_2, spherical microparticles have been obtained. Particles diameter depends on solute concentration in the liquid solution and on the diameter of the injector.

When the process is successful, perfectly spherical particles are formed that are a result of droplets stabilization by surface tension. The visual observation of jet characteristics, the dependence of the particle size on the diameter of the injector, and the perfect spherical shape of the particles are some evidences in favor of a SAS process controlled by the atomization of the liquid solution. Liquid droplets are produced; they are then transformed in spherical particles by solvent elimination due to the very fast mass transfer between the liquid and the supercritical mixture. In the meanwhile, the surface tension zeroes due to the obtainment of near-equilibrium conditions. Therefore, zero or negligible expansion has been observed.

The evolution of particles surface from smooth to rough is relatively simple to be explained, considering that, during the solid formation in the droplet, a crystallization process can superimpose, that tends to create multicrystalline microparticles. They can maintain the spherical shape (or approximately the spherical shape), but a rough surface or a more complex coalescing multicrystal structure can be produced. Crystallization should be particularly fast when the solute is characterized by a very fast crystallization kinetics, due, for example, to a small molecular weight or in the case of a polymer a low molecular weight or a particularly efficient (fast) rearrangement of the polymeric chains.

Nanoparticles

To explain the nanoparticles formation process, two different mechanisms are proposed. In the first case, the droplets are formed; but, the rapid mass transfer of solvent and antisolvent results in high supersaturation of the solute, that causes the formation of several nuclei within the same droplet. The result is the growth of several nanoparticles from one droplet.

The second possible mechanism is that the surface tension between the liquid and the antisolvent disappears at a time scale smaller than the jet break-up of the liquid solution; therefore, no droplets are formed and nucleation and growth of nanoparticles could be the result of gas-like mixing; i.e., gas-to-particle precipitation.

The interface between two miscible fluids at equilibrium at supercritical fluid conditions shows no significant surface tension. But, in the case of the liquid jet injection in the supercritical fluid phase, a time lag exists between the liquid injection and the time at which equilibrium is obtained. The time evolution of the interfacial tension between a liquid and a supercritical fluid has been discussed by Lengsfeld *et al.* [10]. They found that, for the CO_2 + methylene chloride system, at 85 bar and 35°C; i.e., at the complete miscibility conditions, the transient surface tension drops rapidly from approximately 2.5 mN/m at the exit to 0.01 mN/m at about 1 μm from the nozzle tip and the Weber number based approach is no longer applicable.

The literature results are in favour of the gas mixing precipitation mechanism: droplets are not formed at the exit of the injector, the liquid solution is almost instantaneously mixed in the gas phase, from which solids nucleate and eventually grow.

This hypothesis of precipitation mechanism is supported by the following experimental evidences:

The irregular spherical shape of the nanoparticles. If particles are generated from droplets, the surface tension confers them a perfectly spherical shape and the resulting particles obtained by droplet drying will be spherical too. The generation of the nanoparticles from a gaseous phase is compatible, instead, with the irregular shape observed in SEM images (see Figs. **6a** and **6b**).

- As previously discussed, calculations from Lengsfeld *et al.* [10] demonstrated that when SAS process is performed at completely developed supercritical conditions, the time scale of the surface tension disappearance in jets of miscible fluids (solvent and antisolvent) determines the jet evolution as a gas mixing; i.e., no droplets are formed.

- The position of the SAS operating point in the P-x diagram (see the light grey zone in Fig. **8**) is also consistent with the role played by the surface tension in determining or not the formation of droplets. If the surface tension of the liquid injected in the precipitator goes almost instantaneously to zero, no droplets are formed. This process is faster, the more the process conditions are selected at full developed supercritical conditions; i.e., as the pressure increases. As long as the operating point goes to the vicinity of the MCP, this process can compete with the formation of droplets.

- At near critical conditions, equilibrium surface tension disappeared at a time comparable with jet break-up and small droplets can be produced: in this case, the mechanism of powders formation becomes the one droplet – one particle. Therefore, the precipitation process is also regulated by the position of the operating point with respect to MCP.

The nucleation of the solute can superimpose to the diffusion with another characteristic time which depends on various factors also coupled with mass transfer. Chavez *et al.* [19] calculated that two different regimes can be identified. The first one, characterized by slow nucleation and fast diffusion, leads to the formation of particles. The second one, characterized by fast nucleation and slow diffusion, leads to the formation of several nucleation points inside the same droplet and connected nanoparticles surfaces are formed.

REFERENCES

[1]   Reverchon, E. *J. Supercrit. Fluids,* **1999**, 15, 1.
[2]   Shariati, A.; Peters, C.J. *Curr. Opin. Solid State Mater. Sci.,* **2003**, 7, 371.
[3]   Hakuta, Y.; Hayashi, H.; Arai, K.; *Curr. Opin. Solid State Mater. Sci.,* **2003**, 7, 341.
[4]   Knez, Z.; Weidner, E. *Curr. Opin. Solid State Mater. Sci.,* **2003**, 7, 353
[5]   Reverchon, E.; Della Porta, G.; Falivene, M.G. *J. Supercrit. Fluids,* **2000**, 17, 239.
[6]   Reverchon, E.; De Marco, I.; Della Porta, G. *Int. J. Pharm.,* **2002**, 243, 83
[7]   Reverchon, E.; De Marco, I. *J. Supercrit. Fluids,* **2004**, 31, 207.
[8]   Reverchon, E.; De Marco, I. *Powder Technol.,* **2006**, 164, 139.
[9]   Reverchon, E.; De Marco, I.; Torino, E. *J. Supercrit. Fluids,* **2007**, 43, 126.
[10]   Lengsfeld, C.S.; Delplanque, J.P.; Barocas, V.H.; Randolph, T.W. *J. Phys. Chem. B*, **2000**, 104, 2725
[11]   Sarkari, M.; Darrat, I.; Knutson, B.L. *AIChE J.,* **2000**, 46(9), 1850.
[12]   Reverchon, E.; Della Porta, G. *Powder Technol.,* **1999**, 106, 23.
[13]   Adami, R.; Reverchon, E.; Järvenpää, E.; Huopalahti, R. *Powder Technol.,* **2007**, 179, 163.
[14]   Reverchon, E.; Adami, R.; Caputo, G.; De Marco, I. *J. Supercrit. Fluids,* **2008**, 47, 70.
[15]   Reverchon, E.; De Marco, I.; Adami, R.; Caputo, G. *J. Supercrit. Fluids,* **2008**, 44, 98.
[16]   Perez de Diego, Y.; Pellikaan, H.C.; Wubbolts, F.E.; Witkamp, G.J.; Jansens, P.J. *J. Supercrit. Fluids,* **2005**, 35, 147.
[17]   Perez de Diego, Y.; Pellikaan, H.C.; Wubbolts, F.E.; Borchard, G.; Witkamp, G.J.; Jansens, P.J. *J. Supercrit. Fluids,* **2006**, 36, 216.
[18]   Chang S.-C., Lee M.-J., Lin H.-M. The Influence of Phase Behavior on the morphology of protein α-Chymotrypsin prepared via a supercritical anti-solvent process. Proceedings of the 8th International Symposium on Supercritical Fluids; 2006: Kyoto, Japan; paper PB-1-41.pdf.

[19]   Chavez, F.; Debenedetti, P.G.; Luo, J.J.; Dave, R.N.; Pfeffer, R. *Ind. Eng. Chem. Res.*, **2003**, 42, 3156.
[20]   Bouchard, A.; Jovanović, N.; Jiskoot, W.; Mendes, E.; Witkamp, G.-J.; Crommelin, D.J.A.; Hoflanda, G.W. *J. Supercrit. Fluids*, **2007**, 40, 293.
[21]   Werling, J.O.; Debenedetti, P.G. *J. Supercrit. Fluids*, **1999**, 16(2), 167.
[22]   Werling, J.O.; Debenedetti, P.G. *J. Supercrit. Fluids*, **2000**, 18(1), 11.
[23]   Rantakylä, M.; Jäntti, M.; Aaltonen, O.; Hurme, M. *J. Supercrit. Fluids*, **2002**, 24, 251.
[24]   Cocero, M.J.; Ferrero, S. *J. Supercrit. Fluids*, **2002**, 22(3), 237.
[25]   Muhrer, G.; Mazzotti, M.; Müller, M. *J. Supercrit. Fluids*, **2003**, 27, 195.
[26]   Gimeno, M.; Ventosa, N.; Boumghar, Y.; Fournier, J.; Boucher, I.; Veciana, J. *J. Supercrit. Fluids*, **2006**, 38, 94.
[27]   de la Fuente, J.C.; Shariati, A.; Peters, C.J. *J. Supercrit. Fluids*, **2004**, 32, 55.
[28]   Adami, R.; Sesti Osséo, L.; Huopalahti, R.; Reverchon, E. *J. Supercrit. Fluids*, **2007**, 42, 288.
[29]   Reverchon, E.; Caputo, G.; De Marco, I. *Ind. Eng. Chem. Res.*, **2003**, 42, 6406.
[30]   Reverchon, E.; De Marco, I.; Caputo, G.; Della Porta, G. *J. Supercrit. Fluids*, **2003**, 26, 1.
[31]   Reverchon, E.; Adami, R.; De Marco, I.; Laudani, C.G.; Spada, A. *J. Supercrit. Fluids*, **2005**, 35, 76.
[32]   Reverchon, E.; Della Porta, G.; Di Trolio, A.; Pace, S. *Ind. Eng. Chem. Res.*, **1998**, 37, 952.
[33]   Reverchon, E.; Della Porta, G.; Sannino, D.; Ciambelli, P. *Powder Technol.*, **1999**, 102, 127.
[34]   Reverchon, E.; Della Porta, G.; Pallado, P. *Powder Technol.*, **2001**, 114, 17.
[35]   Suo, Q.L.; He, W.Z.; Huang, Y.C.; Huang, C.P.; Li, C.P.; Hong, H.L.; Li, Y.X.; Zhu, M.D., *Powder Technol, .* **2005**, 154, 110.
[36]   Subra, P.; Berroy, P.; Vega, A.; Domingo, C., *Powder Technol.*, **2004**, 142, 13.
[37]   Park, H.J.; Kim, M.-S.; Lee, S.; Kim, J.-S.; Woo, J.-S.; Park, J.-S.; Hwang, S.-J., *Int. J. Pharm.*, **2007**, 328, 152.
[38]   Velaga, S.P.; Ghaderi, R.; Carlfors, J., *Int. J. Pharm.*, **2002**, 231, 155.
[39]   Vatanara, A.; Rouholamini Najafabadi, A.; Gilani, K.; Asgharian, R.; Darabi, M.; Rafiee-Tehrani, M., *J. Supercrit. Fluids*, **2007**, 40, 111.
[40]   Reverchon, E.; De Marco, I. *Powder Technol.*, **2008**, 183, 239.
[41]   Kalogiannis, C.G.; Pavlidou, E.; Panayiotou, C.G. *Ind. Eng. Chem. Res.*, **2005**, 44, 9339.
[42]   Tenorio, A.; Gordillo, M.D.; Pereyra, C.; Martinez de la Ossa, E.J. *J. Supercrit. Fluids*, **2007**, 40, 308.
[43]   Kim, M.-S.; Jin, S.-J.; Kim, J.-S.; Park, H.J.; Song, H.-S.; Neubert R.H.H.; Hwang. S.-J. *Eur. J. Pharm. Biopharm.*, **2008**, 69(2), 454.
[44]   Yeo, S.-D.; Lim, G.-B.; Debenedetti, P.G.; Bernstein, H. *Biotech. Bioeng.*, **1993**, 41, 341.
[45]   Kim, Y.H.; Shing, K.S. *Powder Technol.*, **2007**, 179, 90.
[46]   Kim, Y.H.; Sioutas, C.; Fine, P.; Shing, K.S. *Powder Technol.*, **2008**, 182(3), 354.
[47]   Winters, M.A.; Knutson, B.L.; Debenedetti, P.G.; Sparks, H.G.; Przybycien, T.M.; Stevenson, C.L.; Prestrelski, S.J. *J. Pharm. Sci.*, **1996**, 85(6), 586.
[48]   Moshashaée, S.; Bisrat, M.; Forbes, R.T.; Nyqvist, H.; York, P. *Eur. J. Pharm. Sci.*, **2000**, 11, 239.
[49]   Magnan, C.; Badens, E.; Commenges, N.; Charbit, G. *J. Supercrit. Fluids*, **2000**, 19, 69.
[50]   Caputo, G.; Reverchon, E. *Ind. Eng. Chem. Res.*, **2007**, 46, 4265.
[51]   Reverchon, E.; De Marco, I.; Della Porta, G. *J. Supercrit. Fluids*, **2002**, 23, 81.
[52]   Chang, S.-C.; Lee, M.-J.; Lin, H.-M. *J. Supercrit. Fluids*, **2007**, 40, 420.
[53]   Park, Y.; Curtis, C.W.; Roberts, C.B. *Ind. Eng. Chem. Res.*, **2002**, 41, 1504.
[54]   Bleich, J.; Müller, W B.; Waßmus, W. *Int. J. Pharm.*, **1993**, 97, 111.
[55]   Sousa Costa, M.; Duarte, A.R.C.; Cardoso, M.M.; Duarte, C.M.M. *Int. J. Pharm.*, **2007**, 328, 72.
[56]   Engwicht, A.; Girreser, U.; Müller, B.W. *Int. J. Pharm.*, **1999**, 185, 61.
[57]   Reverchon, E.; Della Porta, G.; De Rosa, I.; Subra, P.; Letourneur, D. *J. Supercrit. Fluids*, **2000**, 18, 239.
[58]   Randolph, T.W.; Randolph, A.D.; Mebes, M.; Yeung S. *Biotechnol. Prog.*, **1993**, 9, 429.
[59]   Sze Tu, L.; Dehghani, F.; Foster, N.R. *Powder Technol.*, **2002**, 126, 134.
[60]   Chen, A.-Z.; Pu, X.-M.; Kang, Y.-Q.; Liao, L.; Yao, Y.-D.; Yin, G.-F. *J. Mater. Sci.: Mater. Med.*, **2007**, 18, 2339.
[61]   Elvassore, N.; Bertucco, A.; Caliceti, P. *Ind. Eng. Chem. Res.*, **2001**, 40, 795.
[62]   Kalogiannis, C.G.; Michailof, C.M.; Panatyiotou, C.G. *Ind. Eng. Chem. Res.*, **2006**, 45, 8738.
[63]   Kim, M.Y.; Lee, Y.W.; Byun, H.-S.; Lim, J.S. *Ind. Eng. Chem. Res.*, **2006**, 45, 3383.
[64]   Taki, S.; Badens, E.; Charbit, G. *J. Supercrit. Fluids*, **2001**, 21, 61.
[65]   Boutin, O.; Maruejouls, C.; Charbit, G. *J. Supercrit. Fluids*, **2007**, 40, 443.
[66]   Carretier, E.; Badens, E.; Guichardon, P.; Boutin, O.; Charbit, G. *Ind. Eng. Chem. Res.*, **2003**, 42, 331.
[67]   Boutin, O.; Badens, E.; Carretier, E.; Charbit, G. *J. Supercrit. Fluids*, **2004**, 31, 89.
[68]   Breitenbach, A.; Mohr, D.; Kissel, T. *J. Control. Release*, **2000**, 63, 53.
[69]   Bitz, C.; Doelker, E., *Int. J. Pharm.*, **1996**, 131, 171.

[70]   Hong, L.; Guo, J.; Gao, Y.; Yuan, W.-K. *Ind. Eng. Chem. Res.*, **2000**, 39, 4882.

[71]   Lefebvre, A.H. In *Atomization and Sprays*; Hemisphere Publishing Corporation: New York, **1989**; pp. 165–222.

[72]   van Konynenburg, P.H.; Scott, R.L. *Philos. Trans. R. Soc. Lond.*, **1980**, 298A, 495.

CHAPTER 4

Particles from Gas-Saturated Solutions and Related Methods for Particle Engineering

A.R. Sampaio de Sousa[1, 2] and Catarina M. M. Duarte[1, 2] *

[1]*Instituto de Tecnologia Química e Biológica, Universidade Nova de Lisboa, Avenida da República, Estação Agronómica Nacional, 2780-157 Oeiras, Portugal and* [2]*Instituto de Biologia Experimental e Tecnológica, Avenida da República, Quinta-do-Marquês, Estação Agronómica Nacional, Apartado 12, 2781-901 Oeiras, Portugal; Email: cduarte@itqb.unl.pt*

Abstract: One of the most promising methods for particle engineering using supercritical fluids is the PGSS – Particles from gas saturated solutions and derived methods. It has been used to micronized drugs and active compounds and to produce composite particles, mainly for pharmaceutical applications, however food applications are starting to arise among experimental work with potential for industrial applications. The morphology and size of the particles obtained is diverse depending on the system used, but they are usually in a micro-nano size range. This chapter presents an overview of the basic principles of the method, several developments that were further undertaken, and a compilation of different examples and systems.

PGSS - BASIC PRINCIPLE

Among the most promising applications of supercritical fluids (SCF), particle engineering processes are now subjected to an escalating interest, since particulate systems with controlled size and morphology can be produced, with the purpose of increasing bio-availability of poorly water soluble molecules, designing sustained and/or targeted-release formulations and modifying the surface properties of particles [1, 2].

Depending on the final purpose, supercritical fluids can be used to produce particles, or to coat existing particles, as means to modify their surface. Either way, there is a chemical and a physical approach to the process. In chemical methods the fluid, is used as a reaction or a deposition medium. When the process involves physical transformations, the existing methods for particle design with supercritical fluids are usually classified upon the role of the fluid in the process.

In PGSS - Particles from Gas-Saturated Solutions, also known as supercritical melt micronization, the supercritical fluid plays a role as a solute, meaning it is dissolved in the bulk of a liquid matrix, either melted compounds or a suspension/solution of the compounds.

This technique was first described by Weidner *et al* [3], and is schematically presented in Figure 1.

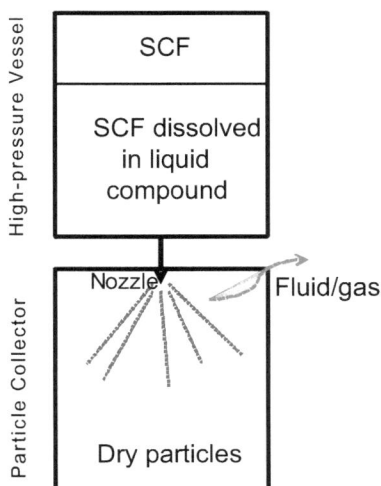

Figure 1: Diagram of PGSS method.

The basic principle of the method relies on the fact that a dense gas (SCF in the Fig. **1**) can be solubilized in large quantities in a liquid (suspension/solution) or a melted solid and the gas-saturated mixture is then rapidly expanded through a nozzle. The expansion of this compressed media causes a temperature drop explained by the Joule-Thomson effect, leading to the complete evaporation of the gas and cooling down of the droplets atomized. The bulk compound(s) solidifies, forming dry particles that are further collected by means of filters, cyclones or other separators.

In what matters the supercritical fluid used, although there are some recent examples of using water [4, 5] and even acetone [6], the most commonly used is carbon dioxide.

The application of this method as opposite to others, where the fluid can act as a solvent or an anti-solvent, mainly lies on these features [adapted from ref. 7]:

-   Low gas demand

-   Low to medium pressure required

-   Absence of organic solvents

-   Small volume of pressurized equipment, facilitating scale-up

-   Small volume of pressurized equipment, facilitating scale-up

-   Large range of materials applicable

-   No solubility requirement of the compounds in the fluid (only of the fluid in the compounds)

On top of that, the solubilization of a gas in a solid matrix is known to lower its viscosity and its melting point, enabling the processing of melted substances at lower temperatures than the ones used in conventional melt techniques. However, depending on the compounds to be precipitated, other methods might fit better the final purpose, and an exhaustive evaluation must be performed before selecting one particular method.

This method in particular is suited for producing micro/nanoparticles for a wide range of applications from pharmaceuticals to food industry. It has been applied not only to the micronization of isolated substances, but also to the co-precipitation of composite particles, either in coating layers or mixed. **Fig. 2** presents some references of examples of micronized systems prepared by PGSS and related methods.

MODELING THE PROCESS

The description of the phenomena that occur in the PGSS process is rather complex and better described by Martin and Cocero in another chapter of this book. It involves a phase change of the gas-saturated solution, from liquid to solid state, as briefly described on the diagram presented in **Figure 2.** When considering solid substances at room temperature, and not solutions as explored in other related methods, this initial liquid state can be achieved at lower temperatures than the ones used without the presence of the fluid, since is lowers the compounds viscosity and reduces the melting point. The reduction range is very wide and can go up to hundreds of degrees difference, depending on the nature of the substances and on the solubility [8] of the fluid in the bulk of the mixture. A typical variation of the melting temperature with pressure is also presented in **Figure 2**.

The parameters to be considered for an exhaustive description of the PGSS process [9-15] include:

-   supercritical fluid thermodynamics,

-   compound's properties,

-   crystallization kinetics (nucleation rate and type),

-   density of the gas-saturated solution (solubilization of the fluid in the bulk mixture), jet/spray (nozzle) hydrodynamics,

-   droplet fluid dynamics,

-   bubble formation and droplet coalescence.

Several kinds of micro- and nanoparticles with different morphologies have been described in literature as obtained by PGSS and related processes, such as spheres, sponges, fibers, porous structures.

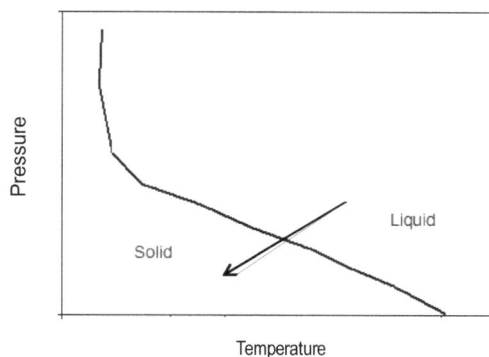

Figure 2: Representation of the phase transition occurring on a PGSS process.

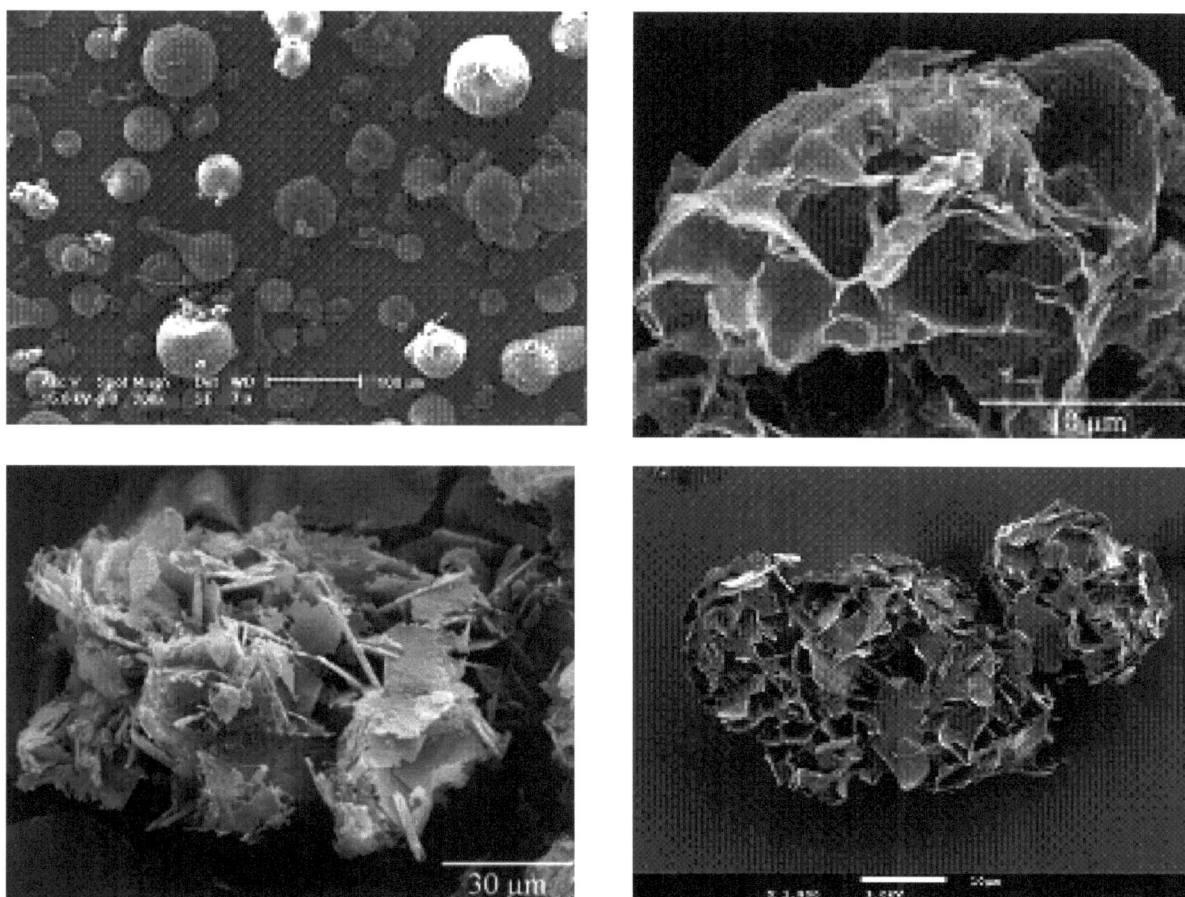

Figure 3: Examples of SEM pictures of particles obtained by PGSS [16].

The influence of the operating conditions (pressure and temperature) was also studied by Kappler et al [17], when the authors performed more than 200 experiments and by statistical evaluation have correlated the size and shape of the particles obtained to a sphericity coefficient to elaborate a predicting model.

RELATED METHODS

Several adaptations have been developed to better adjust this technique to different systems such as dispersions and aqueous solutions.

Concentrated Powder Form

In this process, instead of mixing the substances in a high-pressure stirred vessel, they are blended in a static mixer. The process is called Concentrated Powder Form – CPF [18]. This procedure is used for combining an active substance with a carrier and the mixer allows a better mass transfer.

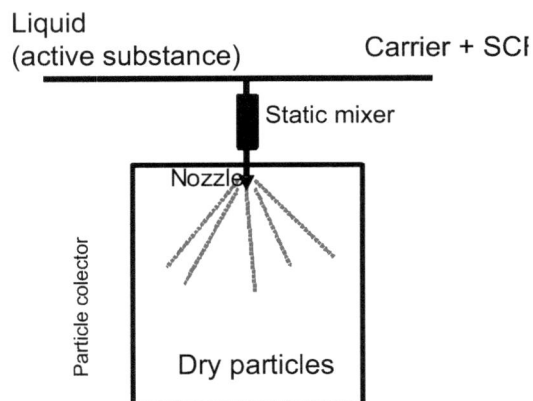

Figure 4: Schematic description of CPF.

Carbon dioxide Assisted Nebulization with Bubble Dryer

In the CAN-BD (Carbon dioxide Assisted Nebulization with Bubble Dryer) [19] method, aqueous solutions and the supercritical fluid are mixed in a low-volume tee with a capillary injector, before depressurization, forming a spray of aerosols.

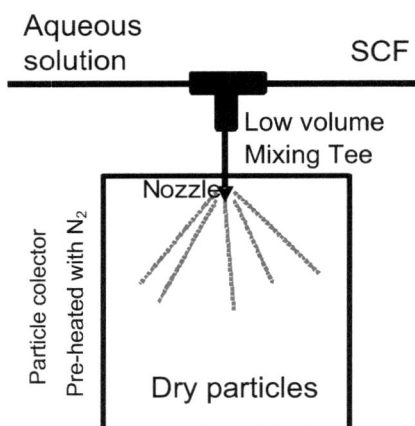

Figure 5: Schematic description of CAN-BD.

Supercritical Assisted Atomization

An improvement to this mixing was later introduced in a process known as SAA (supercritical assisted atomization) [20], where the mixing tee was replaced by a thermostated packed column, to ensure equilibrium conditions. The method is of particularly interest for the development of inhalable powders.

A novel design mixer, i.e., hydrodynamic cavitation mixer was more recently developed by M.-Q. Cai *et al* [21] to improve mass transfer by improving the thermodynamics and hydrodynamics inside the saturator. The feed of the solution and the supercritical fluid to the saturated is made by means of a tee similar to what is used in CAN-BD, and then the saturator holds a cavitation generator inside.

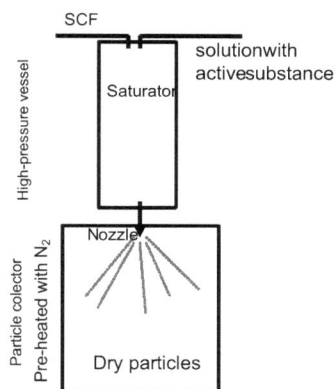

Figure 6: Schematic description of SAA.

Depressurization of an Expanded Liquid Organic Solution

Methods like DELOS (Depressurization of an Expanded Liquid Organic Solution) [22] were developed to enable the processing of gas-saturated mixtures with conventional solvents [23]. In this process an organic solution is mixed with a supercritical fluid and suffers expansion. This mixture is then depressurized through a nozzle, like the previous methods, but the particles are recovered in a filter and the organic solvent is also recovered in a separate vessel.

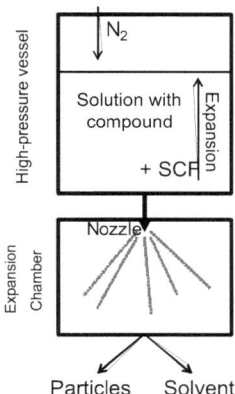

Figure 7: Schematic description of DELOS.

Continuous Powder Coating Spraying Process

The CPCSP [24] has been developed to avoid premature reaction of the carriers of active compounds and allow a continuous PGSS like-process. Therefore, the feed is similar to a CPF process, using a static mixer, but the compounds are added already in a liquefied state.

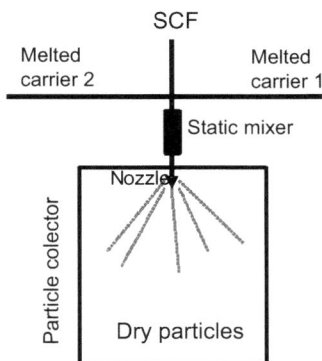

Figure 8: Schematic description of CPCSP.

COMPOUNDS PROCESSED AND PARTICLES OBTAINED

Over the last years, several studies and patents have been published based on this particle formation method, or related processes (SAA, CAN-BD, DELOS, CPF, etc). Although quite a few examples are published as scientific papers applied to polymers, glycerides and pharmaceuticals [2, 23, 25], most of the applications of these methods are patent protected [1], reflecting the feasibility of industrial application of this technique. The particle size and shape is characteristic of each system. A compilation of some representative examples of these publications is summarized in Table **1**:

The design of composite particles as carrier systems of active compounds is a way to achieve more effective therapeutics, to mask unpleasant tastes, to protect ingredients, or even to enable the incorporation of the active compound in an incompatible matrix.

In this chapter three illustrative examples of lipid particles with active compounds, formed by PGSS, are presented: trans-chalcone was used and tested as pharmaceutical example [78]; caffeine was studied for incorporation in cosmetic/dermal products [76]; and mixtures of natural antioxidants were included in lipid particles for food applications [16]. Each of these examples was tested according to the final purpose. Preliminary tests are also described for the incorporation in lipid carriers of an aroma fraction, recovered from wine waste products [16].

Table 1: Compilation of representative examples of products processed by PGSS and related processes.

Compound	References
Adhesives	26
Benzoic acid, glucose	27
Glycerides	10, 12, 25, 28, 29
Metal oxides	19, 27
Phosphors	30
Plastic additives	31
Polymers	17, 32-37
Powder coating	38, 39
Powder lacquer	40
Albuterol sulfate	27, 41
Cromolyn sodium	27, 41
Na_2Fe (DTPA)	42
Antibiotics	27, 43-47
Cyclodextrins	48
Cyclodextrins + active compounds	49-51
Felodipine	52
Steroids	53, 54
Griseofulvin	55, 56
Riboflavine	57
Sodium and ammonium chloride	58
Terbutaline	59
Vaccines	60
Spinels	61
Enzymes	19, 62
DL- alanine	42
Nifedipine	7, 63
Zirconyl nitrate hydrate	64
Chitosan	44, 65
Polymers + protein	66-68
Polymers+active compound	52, 69
Cyclosporine	70

Table 1: cont...

Colourants	22, 71
Citrus flavour	72
Potassium iodide	58
Lipid + protein	73, 74
Lipid + active compound	75-78
Anthocyanins	79
Cefadroxil	80

PHARMACEUTICAL APPLICATIONS

Trans-chalcone, is the core structure of a wider group natural occurring substances, whose properties have been studied for a large range of pharmacological activities.

Particles of trans-chalcone alone and with different carriers were produced using the PGSS technique. Table **2** summarizes the formulations prepared.

Table 2: Summary of chalcone + carrier formulations.

#	Carrier	Composition
A	-	-
B	Gelucire 50/13	1: 1
C	Precirol ato5	1: 1
D	Gelucire 50/13 + Precirol ato5	2: 1: 1

After 12 hours of immersion in different simulated fluids the concentration of chalcone in solution was determined and the results are presented on Fig. **9**.

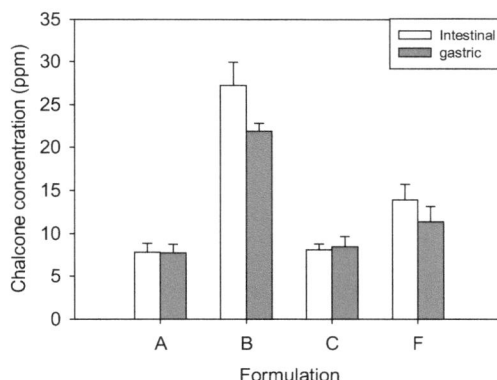

Figure 9: Concentration of trans-chalcone in gastric (grey) and intestinal (white) simulated fluids for the formulations A, B, C and D.

Results show that the maximum amount of micronized chalcone (A) solubilized both in gastric and intestinal simulated fluids was about 8 ppm, as well as for formulation C (chalcone + precirol). Formulation B (chalcone + gelucire) however, was able to increase the concentration in the gastric and intestinal fluids up to 22 ppm and 27 ppm, respectively. The formulation containing both gelucire and precirol lead to an intermediate value between these two cases and the solubilized chalcone was 12 ppm for gastric fluid and 14 ppm intestinal fluid.

These results suggest that the nature of the carrier has a significant effect on the dissolution of the active compounds. The hydrophilic nature of Gelucire 50/13 enabled the formation of smaller and more homogeneous particles that lead to an enhanced solubility of chalcone.

COSMETICAL APPLICATIONS

Caffeine was selected as model active compound for being a hydrophilic substance, and thus a challenge to incorporate in lipid carriers, and also because of its therapeutical and cosmetical applications, namely in the anti-cellulite activity, by stimulation of fat metabolism [81]. Lumulse™ GMS K was elected as lipid carrier, since it can be used as a surfactant broadening the possibilities of attachment to caffeine.

A formulation of GMS + caffeine (10: 2 mass proportion) and caffeine as supplied, were separately incorporated in a gel (o/w emulsion – Simulgel™ 600 PHA, Seppic) with 5% caffeine content in the final product. The prepared gels were homogenized and its final appearance was a viscous suspension of white particles and a white paste, for caffeine and for the formulation, respectively.

The gels obtained were tested for caffeine release and permeability through a membrane using a Franz-cell *in vitro* test (Fig. **10**). This cell consists of a two compartment glass vessel, separated by a membrane. The acceptor compartment (below) was filled with a PBS (phosphate buffer solution, pH 7, 4), which is stirred and thermostatized (at 32°C as reference temperature for human skin). In the donor compartment (above) a dose of the gel was added (large enough to ensure constant concentration during the experiment), and aliquots (350μL) of the receptor fluid were collected at given times to follow the diffusion rate of the compound. The membrane used, cellulose acetate (Sartorius, pore size 0, 2 μm), is not the best option to mimetize human skin [82], however, it is commonly used for preliminary *in vitro* tests [83, 84]. To ensure hydration, the membrane was previously soaked in PBS for 30 minutes.

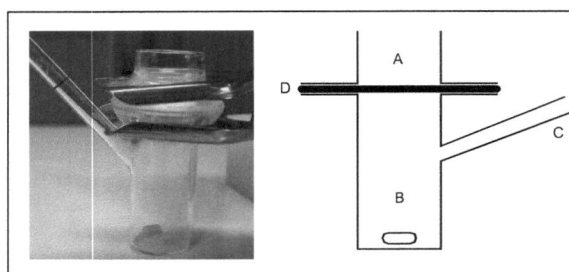

Figure 10: Franz-cell used for the release of caffeine from a gel through a membrane. (A) donor compartment, (B) stirred receptor fluid, (C) sampling port, (D) membrane.

The amount of caffeine in the aliquots was determined by HPLC-DAD analysis.

Fig. **11** presents the diffusion results through a cellulose acetate membrane for the gels with caffeine and with caffeine-loaded lipid particles. The latter showed a much slower and controlled release, without an initial burst validating the possibility of using GMS particles as controlled release agents for cosmetical applications.

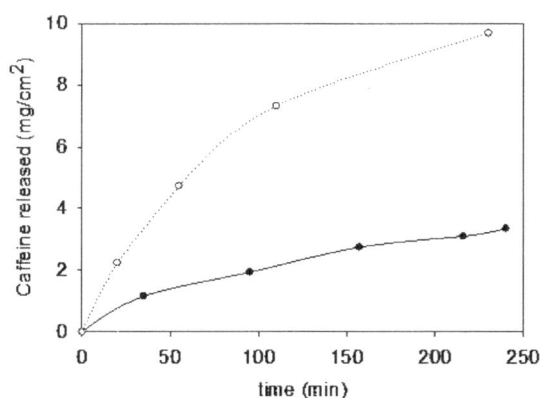

Figure 11: Release profiles of caffeine obtained for the different gels: (dashed line) caffeine alone, (full line) formulation B.

NUTRACEUTICAL APPLICATION

Vegetable oils are regarded as a good source of polyunsaturated fatty acids (PUFA's) in the diet, especially when compared to animal fats, however the PUFA's aren't just responsible for the nutritional value of the oil, they are also responsible for their instability. Exposure to air, heat, light and moisture, enhances the chemical reactivity of the double bonds which will oxidize and form radicals that will lead to deterioration of the oil. In recent years the stabilization of edible oils has been investigated by several research groups, and one of the most promising ways to achieve it is the addition of natural antioxidants. [85-88]

This study presents a different approach to the addition of natural antioxidants to edible oils, namely sunflower oil, the most widely produced in Europe. Lipid particles (Precirol ato 5 and Lumulse GMS K 50: 50) were produced to enclosure different natural antioxidants such as tocopherols, ascorbic acid, phytosterols and polyphenolic compounds (extracted from olive residues), which represent some of the most studied families of antioxidants. The particles obtained were then incorporated in sunflower oil and its stability was evaluated through tests of acidity. The formulations studied were (A) – ascorbic acid (17%); (B) – ascorbic acid (17%) + tocopherols (2%); (C) – ascorbic acid (17%) + phytosterols (5%); (D) ascorbic acid (33%); (E) – ascorbic acid (17%) + phytosterols (5%) + anticaking agent (6%); (F) – Natural extract (15%); control - sunflower oil with lipid particles without antixiodants. The acidity tests, measuring the percentage of free fatty acids (% FFA) expressed in oleic acid percentage, were performed according to IUPAC standard methods (2.201, 1987), and consist of a titulation of the free fatty acids with an ethanolic solution of potassium hydroxide. Results are presented in Fig. **12**.

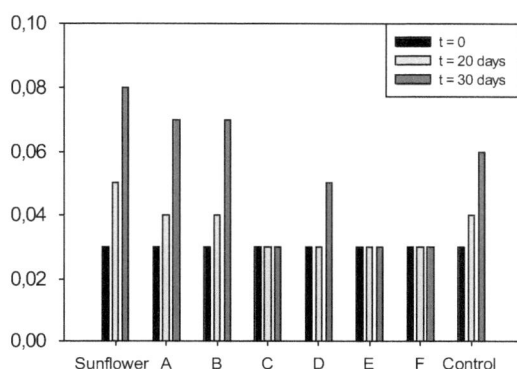

Figure 12: Results of the oxidative stability tests, %FFA (oleic acid %).

Ascorbic acid alone (A and D) demonstrated to have already some effect decreasing %FFA and peroxide values at a concentration of 17%, but only at a concentration of 33% the steadiness of the original %FFA was kept up to 20 days. Formulation B (with 2% tocopherols) did not present significant changes when compared to formulation A. Phytosterols and ascorbic acid together (C and E) tend to reduce the %FFA. The presence of the anticaking agent (E) showed an even greater effect in the peroxide value and induction time.

The addition of lipid microparticles alone (control sample) enhanced the oxidative resistance at low temperature, with a decrease in the %FFA as compared to the original oil.

The microparticles with the natural extract (F) presented the overall highest oxidative stability as the free fatty acid percentage was maintained at the initial reference values of sunflower oil. This happens because the natural extract is a complex mixture of phenolic compounds interacting synergistically between them.

Table 3: Amounts of the aromatic compound present in the feed and recovery percentages (EAC – ethyl acetate, IBUT – isobuthyl alcohol, IAC – isoamyl acetate, EHEX – ethyl hexanoate, HAC – hexyl acetate, 1-HEX - hexanol, LIN – linalool)

Aroma compounds	EAC	IBUT	IAC	IAM	EHEX	HAC	1-HEX	LIN
Feed concentration (ppm)	6422, 9	824, 4	2170, 4	365, 3	2237, 4	2159, 5	754, 2	881, 7
% recovered in particles	-	19, 7	6, 5	16, 0	6, 4	13, 6	54, 0	71, 5

AROMA ENCAPSULATION

Fragrances and flavours are part of an ever growing industry parallel to food, cosmetics and toiletries, pharmaceuticals, detergents and other applications which include candles, air fresheners, aromatherapy and pesticides.

These compounds are extremely volatile and usually sensitive to oxidation. Encapsulation of aromatic compounds can minimize these issues by avoiding undesirable molecular interactions and protecting against light-induced reactions, which result in a longer retention of the compound in the final product, even allowing a controlled release.

The carriers elected were, similarly to what was used in the previous example, a mixture of Precirol ato 5 and Lumulse GMS K (50: 50), and the aroma fraction represented 25 wt% of the total feed. This fraction is mainly composed of ethanol (47, 7 wt%) and water with the aromatic compounds, described in Table **3**.

At first sight, the recovery percentages of the aromatic compounds entrapped in the lipid particles are low, with exception to linalool. These results are due to the higher volatility of the smaller compounds, which increases in contact with carbon dioxide and with temperature (which was set at 325 K). When taking into account the high ethanol content (47, 7 wt%) of the feed aroma fraction, acting as a preferential co-solvent to solubilize the compounds in the gas phase, and the fact that the compounds are water soluble in opposition to the lipophilic carriers, the results go from weak to promising.

Some alternative options have been proposed to increase the recovery percentages of the aromas. These include the usage of a carrier with a higher hydrophilic-lipophilic balance (HLB), enhancing the aroma-carrier affinity; the decrease in stirring time during the PGSS processing, the increase in concentration of the initial aroma fraction and respective decrease of ethanol content, to minimize the solubilization of the aromas in the gas phase. Parallel stability studies of moisture content and aroma composition in the particles with time should also be accessed.

These results show that indeed lipid particles processed by PGSS have the potential to encapsulate aromas.

CONCLUSIONS

The PGSS technique might have a prominent role in the future of drug delivery especially for the preparation of microparticulate systems. In fact several industrial plants are already running with capacities of some hundred kilograms per hour (Natex, Austria, Thar Technologies, USA, Uhde HPT). [89]

With the rising interest of scientists, companies and number of patents being submitted it is unquestionable the potential of supercritical fluids as a means for particle engineering, PGSS related methods in particular, especially considering they can comply with green chemistry principles and GMP conditions [90]. Innovations and improvements to the existing techniques are being continuously studied and future development points to the coupling of the particle design processes with other existing methods such as synthesis/ reaction [91] and extraction.

REFERENCES

[1]   J. Jung, M. Perrut, *J Supercriti Fluids*, **2001**. 20(3): p. 179-219.
[2]   M. Bahrami, S. Ranjbarian, *J Supercrit Fluids*, **2007**. 40(2): p. 263-283.
[3]   E. Weidner, Z. Knez, Z. Novak, Patent WO9521688, **1995**
[4]   C. B. Xu, A. S. Teja, *J Supercrit Fluids*, **2006**, 39(1): p. 135-141.
[5]   Z. Fang, H. Assaaoudi, H. B. Lin, X. M. Wang, I. S. Butler, J. A. Kozinski, *J Nanoparticle Research*, **2007**, 9(4): p. 683-687.
[6]   M. Moner-Girona, A. Roig, E. Molins, J. Llibre, *J Sol-Gel Sci Techn*, **2003**. 26(1): p. 645-649.
[7]   E. Weidner, Z. Knez, Z. Novak, in: G. Brunner, M. Perrut (Eds.), Proceedings for the Third International Symposium for Supercritical Fluids, vol. 3, **1994**, p. 229.
[8]   P.G. Jessop, B. Subramaniam, *Chem. Rev.*, **2007**, 107, p.2666-2694
[9]   M. Strumendo, A. Bertucco, N. Elvassore, *J Supercrit Fluids*, **2007** 41(1): p. 115-125
[10]   J. Li, M. Rodrigues, A. Paiva, H. A. Matos, E. G. de Azevedo, *Aiche Journal*, **2005**. 51(8): p. 2343-2357.
[11]   J. Li, H.A. Matos, E.G. de Azevedo, *J. Supercrit. Fluids*, **2004**, 32, p. 275–286.
[12]   M. Calderone, E. Rodier, J. J. Letourneau, J. Fages, *J Supercrit Fluids*, **2007**. 42(2): p. 189-199.
[13]   Martín, M.J. Cocero, *Advanced Drug Delivery Reviews*, **2008**, 60(3), p. 339-350
[14]   M. J. Cocero, Á. Martín, F. Mattea, S. Varona, *J Supercrit Fluids*, **2009**, 47(3), p. 546-555
[15]   N. Elvassore, M. Flaibani, A. Bertucco, P. Caliceti, *Ind. Eng. Chem. Res*, **2003**, 42, p. 5924–5930.
[16]   A.R.Sampaio de Sousa, Developemnt of functional particles sign supercritical fluid technology, Thesis, **2007**
[17]   P. Kappler, W. Leiner, M. Petermann, E. Weidner, in 6th International Symposium on Supercritical Fluids, **2003**, Versailles, France.

[18]   Weinreich, R. Steiner, E. Weidner, J. Dirscherl, Patent WO99/17868, **1999**

[19]   R. E. Sievers, U. Karst, P. D. Milewski, S. P. Sellers, B. A. Miles, J. D. Schaefer, C. R. Stoldt, C. Y. Xu, *Aerosol Science and Technology*, **1999,** 30(1), p. 3-15.

[20]   E. Reverchon, *Ind Eng Chem Res*, **2002**, 41(10), p. 2405-2411.

[21]   Mei-Qiang Cai, Yi-Xin Guan, Shan-Jing Yao, Zi-Qiang Zhu, *J Supercrit Fluids*, **2008**, 43(3), p. 524-534

[22]   N. Ventosa, S. Sala, J. Veciana, J. Torres, J. Llibre, *Crystal Growth & Design*, **2001,** 1(4), p. 299-303.

[23]   A. Shariati, C. J. Peters, *Curr Op Solid State Mater Sci*, **2003**, 7(4-5), p. 371-383.

[24]   E. Weidner, M. Petermann, K. Blatter, V. Rekowski, *Chem Eng Techn*, **2001,** 24(5), p. 529-533.

[25]   Z. Knez, E. Weidner, in High pressure process technology: fundamentals and applications, A. Bertucco and G. Vetter, Editors. **2001**, Elsevier. p. 587-611.

[26]   T.A. Cole, K.A. Nielsen, Patent US5066522, **1989**

[27]   R.E. Sievers, B.A. Miles, S.P. Sellers, P.D. Milewski, K.D. Kusek, P.G. Klutez., in Respiratory Drug Delivery IV Conference. **1998**. South Carolina, USA

[28]   Z. Novak, P. Senvar-Bozic, A. Rizner, Z. Knez, in Fluidi Supercritici e Loro Applicazioni. **1993**. Ravello, Italy.

[29]   P. Munuklu, P. J. Jansens, *J Supercrit Fluids*, **2007,** 40(3), p. 433-442.

[30]   Y. Xu, B. A. Watkins, R. E. Sievers, X. P. Jing, P. Trowga, C. S. Gibbons, A. Vecht, *Applied Physics Letters*, **1997**, 71(12), p. 1643-1645.

[31]   W.D. Prince, G.E. Keller, W.A. Fraser, P.S. Leung, Patent EP0590647, **1993**

[32]   Weidner, R. Steiner, Z. Knez, in High Pressure Chemical Engineering, P.R. von Rohr and C. Trepp, Editors. **1996,** Elsevier Science.

[33]   J. Y. Hao, M. J. Whitaker, G. Serhatkulu, K. M. Shakesheff, S. M. Howdle, *J Mater Chem*, **2005**, 15(11), p. 1148-1153.

[34]   Z. Knez, in 6th International Symposium on Supercritical Fluids. **2003**. Versailles, France.

[35]   Reverchon, A. Antonacci, *J Supercrit Fluids*, **2007,** 39(3), p. 444-452.

[36]   S. P. Nalawade, L.P.B.M. Janssen, in 6th International Symposium on Supercritical Fluids. **2003**. Versailles, France.

[37]   S. P. Nalawade, F. Picchioni, Lpbm Janssen, *Chem Eng Sci*, **2007,** 62(6), p. 1712-1720.

[38]   Mandel, in 4th International Symposium on Supercritical Fluids. **1997**. Sendai, Japan.

[39]   E. Weidner, M. Petermann, K. Blatter, H.U. Simmrock, in 6th Meeting on Supercritical Fluids, **1999,** Nottingham, UK.

[40]   M. Kieser, O. Stahlecker, Patente DE19707051, **1998**

[41]   R. E. Sievers, P.D. Milewski, S.P. Sellers, B.A. Miles, B.J. Korte, K.D. Kusek, G.S. Clark, B. Mioskowski, J.A. Villa, in 5th International Symposium on Supercritical Fluids. **2000**. Atlanta, USA.

[42]   R. E. Sievers, U. Karst, Patent EP0677332, **1995**

[43]   E. Reverchon, G. Della Porta, *Pure and Applied Chemistry*, **2001**, 73(8), p. 1293-1297.

[44]   E. Reverchon, A. Antonacci, *Biotech Bioeng*, **2007,** 97(6), p. 1626-1637.

[45]   E. Reverchon, A. Spada, *Powder Technology*, **2004**. 141(1-2), p. 100-108.

[46]   E. Reverchon, G. Della Porta, *J Supercrit Fluids*, **2003**. 26(3): p. 243-252.

[47]   E. Reverchon, G. Della Porta, A. Spada, *J Pharm Pharmacol*, **2003**. 55(11), p. 1465-1471.

[48]   E. Reverchon, A. Antonacci, *Biotech Bioeng*, **2006**. 94(4): p. 753-761.

[49]   T. Van Hees, G. Piel, B. Evrard, X. Otte, L. Thunus, L. Delattre, *Pharm Res*, **1999**. 16(12): p. 1864-1870.

[50]   M. Charoenchaitrakool, F. Dehghani, N. R. Foster, *Int J Pharm*, **2002**. 239(1-2): p. 103-112.

[51]   B. Marongiu, A. Piras, S. Porcedda, A. Lai, S. Lai, E. Locci. in 6th International Symposium on Supercritical Fluids. **2003**. Versailles, France.

[52]   J. Kerc, S. Srcic, Z. Knez, P. Sencar-Bozic, *Int J Pharm*, **1999**. 182(1): p. 33-39.

[53]   Della Porta, S. F. Ercolino, L. Parente, E. Reverchon, *J Pharm Sci*, **2006**. 95(9): p. 2062-2076.

[54]   R. E. Sievers, E. T. S. Huang, J. A. Villa, G. Engling, P. R. Brauer, *J Supercrit Fluids*, **2003**. 26(1): p. 9-16.

[55]   Della Porta, C. De Vittori, E. Reverchon, *Aaps Pharmscitech*, **2005**. 6(3).

[56]   E. Reverchon, G. Della Porta, A. Spada, A. Antonacci, *J Pharm Pharmacol*, **2004**. 56(11): p. 1379-1387

[57]   F. Otto, S. Gruner, B. Weinreich. in 6th International Symposium on Supercritical Fluids. **2003**. Versailles, France.

[58]   E. Reverchon, A. Spada, *Ind Eng Chem Res*, **2004**. 43(6): p. 1460-1465.

[59]   E. Reverchon, G. Della Porta, *Int J Pharm*, **2003**. 258(1-2), p. 1-9.

[60]   R. E. Sievers, B. P. Quinn, S. P. Cape, J. A. Searles, C. S. Braun, P. Bhagwat, L. G. Rebits, D. H. McAdams, J. L. Burger, J. A. Best, L. Lindsay, M. T. Hernandez, K. O. Kisich, T. Iacovangelo, D. Kristensen, D. Chen, *J Supercrit Fluids*, **2007**. 42(3): p. 385-391

[61]   C. Y. Xu, R. E. Sievers, U. Karst, B. A. Watkins, C.M. Karbiwnyk, W.C. Andersen, J.D. Schaefer, C.R. Stoldt, in Green Chemistry: Frontiers in Benign Chemical Synthesis and Processes, P.T. Anastas and T.C. Williamson, Editors. **1998**, Oxford University Press: Oxford. p. 313-335.

[62]   S. P. Sellers, G. S. Clark, R. E. Sievers, J. F. Carpenter, *J Pharm Sci*, **2001**. 90(6): p. 785-797

[63]   P. SencarBozic, S. Srcic, Z. Knez, J. Kerc, *Int J Pharm*, **1997**. 148(2): p. 123-130.

[64]   E. Reverchon, R. Adami, G. Caputo, *J Supercrit Fluids*, **2006**. 37(3): p. 298-306.

[65]   E. Reverchon, A. Antonacci, *Ind Eng Chem Res*, **2006**. 45(16): p. 5722-5728.

[66]   M.S. Watson, M.J. Whitaker, S.M. Howdle, K.M. Shakesheff, *Advanced Materials*, **2002**. 14(24): p. 1802-1804.

[67]   S.M. Howdle, M.S. Watson, M.J. Whitaker, V.K. Popov, M.C. Davies, F.S. Mandel, J.D. Wang, K.M. Shakesheff, *Chem. Commun.*, **2001**, p. 109-110.

[68]   M. J. Whitaker, J. Y. Hao, O. R. Davies, G. Serhatkulu, S. Stolnik-Trenkic, S. M. Howdle, K. M. Shakesheff, *J Control Release*, **2005**. 101(1-3): p. 85-92.

[69]   S. Suttiruengwong, J. Rolker, I. Smirnova, W. Arlt, M. Seiler, L. Luderitz, Y. P. de Diego, P. J. Jansens, *Pharm Develop Techn*, **2006**. 11(1): p. 55-70.

[70]   A. Tandya, F. Dehghani, N. R. Foster, *J Supercrit Fluids*, **2006**. 37(3): p. 272-278.

[71]   E. Reverchon, R. Adami, I. De Marco, C. G. Laudani, A. Spada, *J Supercrit Fluids*, **2005**. 35(1): p. 76-82.

[72]   S. Gruner, F. Otto, B. Weinreich. in 6th International Symposium on Supercritical Fluids. **2003**. Versailless, France.

[73]   P. Caliceti, A. Brossa, S. Salmaso, S. Bersani, N. Elvassore, A. Bertucco. in Intern. Symp. Control. Rel. Bioact. Mater. **2006**.

[74]   S. Salmaso, S. Bersani, N. Elvassore, A. Bertucco, P.Caliceti, *Int J Pharm*, In Press

[75]   M. Calderone, E. Rodier, J. Fages, *Particulate Sci Techn*, **2007**. 25(3): p. 213-225.

[76]   A.R. Sampaio de Sousa, Ana Luisa Simplicio, Herminio C. de Sousa, Catarina M.M. Duarte, *J Supercrit Fluids*, **2007**. 43(1): p. 120-125.

[77]   M. Rodrigues, N. Peirico, H. Matos, E. G. de Azevedo, M. R. Lobato, A. J. Almeida, *J Supercrit Fluids*, **2004**. 29(1-2): p. 175-184.

[78]   A.R. Sampaio de Sousa, R. Silva, F. H. Tay, A.L. Simplício, S.G. Kazarian, C. M.M. Duarte, *J Supercrit Fluids*, **2009**, 48(2), 120-125

[79]   T.Vatai, M. Škerget, Ž. Knez, S. Kareth, M.Wehowski, E. Weidner, *J Supercrit Fluids*, **2008**, 45(1), p.32-36

[80]   L. Zhiyi, J. Jingzhi, L. Xuewu, T. Huihua, W. Wei, *J Supercrit Fluids*, **2009**, 48(3), p.247-252

[81]   C. Bertin, H. Zunino, J. C. Pittet, P. Beau, P. Pineau, M. Massonneau, C. Robert, J. Hopkins, *J Cosmetic Sci*, **2001**. 52(4): p. 199-210.

[82]   M. Dias, A. Farinha, E. Faustino, J. Hadgraft, J. Pais, C. Toscano, *Int J Pharm*, **1999**. 182(1): p. 41-47.

[83]   Herai, T. Gratieri, J. A. Thomazine, Mvlb Bentley, R. F. V. Lopez, *Int J Pharm*, **2007**. 329(1-2): p. 88-93.

[84]   E. B. Souto, R. H. Muller, *Pharmazie*, **2007**. 62(7): p. 505-509.

[85]   S. Naz, R. Siddiqi, H. Sheikh, S. A. Sayeed, *Food Research International*, **2005**. 38(2): p. 127-134.

[86]   N. V. Yanishlieva, E. M. Marinova, *Eur J Lipid Sci Techn*, **2001**. 103(11): p. 752-767.

[87]   M. Van Aardt, S. E. Duncan, T. E. Long, S. F. O'Keefe, J. E. Marcy, S. R. Sims, *J Agri Food Chem*, **2004**. 52(3): p. 587-591.

[88]   C. Gertz, *Eur J Lipid Sci Techn*, **2004**. 106(11): p. 736-745.

[89]   I.Pasquali, R. Bettini, *Int J Pharm*, **2008**, 364(2), p. 176-187

[90]   C. Vemavarapu, M. J. Mollan, M. Lodaya, T. E. Needham, *Int J Pharm*, **2005**. 292(1-2): p. 1-16.

[91]   L. Owens, K. S. Anseth, T. W. Randolph, *Macromolecules*, **2002**. 35(11), p. 4289-4296.

CHAPTER 5

Fundamentals and Modeling of Supercritical Precipitation Processes

Ángel Martín* and María José Cocero

High Pressure Processes Group. Department of Chemical Engineering and Environmental Technology. Faculty of Science. Prado de la Magdalena s/n 47011 Valladolid (Spain); Email: mamaan@iq.uva.es

Abstract: Precipitation processes based on the use of supercritical fluids have undergone considerable development during the last years. One of the main pending tasks at this moment is the development of a systematic procedure for the design and scale-up of these processes. This requires not only empirical knowledge, but also information about the fundamentals of the process. This work aims to review the published literature dealing with a fundamental investigation and modeling of supercritical fluid precipitation processes.

INTRODUCTION

Precipitation processes in general and supercritical precipitation processes in particular involve several simultaneous phenomena that interact in a very complex way: the formation and growth of particle nuclei, the mixing between different substances through mass transfer or fluid mechanic processes, etc. For controlling these processes, it is usually possible to manipulate several parameters (temperature, pressure, composition, geometric design...). However, very often these process parameters have a simultaneous influence on several aspects of the precipitation process: for example, temperature simultaneously affects the rates of particle formation and growth, as well as the volumetric and transport properties of the fluid and therefore the mass transfer and flow processes. Obviously, this makes very difficult to know *a priori* the effect of a modification in a certain process parameter. Moreover, and depending on the application, different objectives are pursued with the precipitation: the production of particles of a specific size and shape, the formation of composites with a certain composition and structure, the production of a formulation with specific organoleptic properties, etc., and the different process parameters can influence these properties in different ways that are also difficult to predict. A purely empirical or statistical analysis of the influence of different process parameters on these characteristics can be very useful or even compulsory, especially during the first stages of the development of a certain application. But if a detailed knowledge of the process is to be obtained in order to propose a optimization and scale-up for a commercial application, and to be able to achieve the robust and reproducible performance required by the regulatory agencies, it is necessary to have a deeper knowledge and understanding of what is happening during the precipitation process and of its fundamentals. Mechanistic mathematical models based on experimental evidence are a very useful tool for this purpose, because they provide additional information that complement experimental data, providing insight into some aspects of the process that are very difficult to study only with experiments. Being precipitation processes with supercritical fluids a relatively mature technology, some mathematical models of these processes have been already proposed [1]. In this chapter, the key aspects of these models are described.

Solubility and Supersaturation

The driving force for a precipitation is the departure from the equilibrium conditions. This departure can be quantified by the supersaturation S, defined as the ratio between the concentration of the solute in the fluid y and the equilibrium concentration y^{eq}, as presented in Eq. (1):

$$S = y/y^{eq} \qquad (1)$$

As it will be shown later, the rate of different stages of the precipitation is a strong function of the supersaturation. Therefore, an accurate calculation of the equilibrium concentration of the solid in the supercritical fluid is essential for the modelling of the precipitation process.

The experimental determination or calculation of the solubility of solids in supercritical fluids is also of interest for developing other applications of supercritical fluid technology, as for example extractions or fractionations. For this reason, these aspects are relatively well known and several calculation procedures have been proposed. These methods can be classified into two main categories: empirical correlations and Equation of State (EoS)-based calculations.

Ana Rita C. Duarte & Catarina M. M. Duarte (Eds)

The empirical equation which is most frequently used to correlate solubility is Chrastil equation [2]. This equation proposes to calculate the solubility as a function of the density of the supercritical fluid, as shown in Eq. (2):

$$\ln(y_{eq}) = k \cdot \ln(\rho_{SCF}) + \alpha/T + \beta \qquad (2)$$

Where k is the association number, α depends on the heat of solvation and the heat of vaporization of the solute and β depends on its molecular weight. This equation is a mere correlation tool and experimental data is required in order to calculate its parameters. In principle, this equation is only suitable to describe the solubility in pure supercritical fluids, but Sauceau *et al.* [3] presented a modification of this equation that can be applied to systems with co-solvents, calculating the association number k as the sum of two contributions $k_1 + k_2$, which are related to the supercritical fluid and the co-solvent, respectively.

Equation of State-based models have a more solid theoretical background, but to apply them it is necessary to have more information about the physical properties of the solid. These models are based on solving the condition of equality of the fugacity in the different phases (Eq. 3):

$$
\begin{aligned}
f_{SCF}^{L} &= f_{SCF}^{V} \\
f_{CS}^{L} &= f_{CS}^{V} \\
f_{S}^{S} &= f_{S}^{L} = f_{S}^{V}
\end{aligned}
\qquad (3)
$$

Since most Equations of State cannot describe the fugacity of solid phases, an approximation is necessary to calculate this fugacity. Two different approximations have been proposed. In the first one, originally proposed by McHugh *et al.* [4], the sublimation pressure of the solid is used as reference to calculate the fugacity of the solid, Eq. (4). In the second one, proposed by Kikic *et al.* [5], the fugacity of the solid is calculated as a function of the fugacity of a hypothetical subcooled liquid as in Eq. (5).

$$f^{S}(P,T) = P^{sub}(T)\phi^{sub}\exp\left[v^{s}\left(\frac{P - P^{sub}(T)}{RT}\right)\right] \qquad (4)$$

$$f^{S}(P,T) = f^{L}(P,T)\exp\left\{\frac{\left(v^{S} - v^{L}\right)}{RT} + \left[\frac{\Delta H^{fus}}{RT^{fus}}\left(1 - \frac{T^{fus}}{T}\right)\right]\right\} \qquad (5)$$

Both approaches are in principle equally valid for the calculation of the solubilities, being the main and most obvious difference between them the different physical properties required to apply them: the sublimation pressure in the first case, and the temperature and enthalpy of fusion in the second case. Therefore the main aspect that has to be considered in order to decide which of the two approaches is the most suitable for a certain application, is the availability of these physical properties. Nevertheless, in certain cases there are differences in the performance of the calculations with the two approaches. In particular, in applications like the correlation of the melting temperature of a solid submerged in a supercritical fluid, Eq. (5) can show a better performance because it implements the normal melting temperature of the substance as an input parameter [6].

Besides the physical properties that appear in Eqs. (4) and (5), the properties required by the Equation of State used to calculate fugacities are also required to apply the Equation of State-based approach. The most frequent selection is a cubic equation of state such as Peng-Robinson, Soave-Redlich-Kwong or Patel-Teja. In these cases, the critical properties are required, which may pose a problem when these properties not only are not known, but also have little physical sense as in the case of applications with polymers. If the critical properties cannot be experimentally determined, several group-contribution methods are available to estimate it. Two of the most frequently used the Joback method [7] and the Constantinou-Gani method [8].

Several non-cubic Equations of State are also available and have been used to describe systems with supercritical fluids. Some examples are:

- The Perturbed Hard-Sphere-Chain (PHSC) Equation of State and related equations [9]: this equation, presented in Eq. 6, describes molecules as a chain of hard spheres, which are characterized by the number of hard spheres per molecule r, the hard sphere diameter σ and the minimum energy in the pair potential ε. This equation is particularly suitable to describe systems with polymers or other high molecular weight substances, because the three parameters r, σ and ε allow a physically reasonable characterization of these molecules. Colussi et al [10] presented a comparison of the performance of three different EoS (Sanchez-Lacombe, Peng-Robinson and PHSC) in different phase equilibrium calculations with supercritical fluids, concluding that the PHSC EoS showed advantages in the calculations of the solubility of solids or with complex molecules as for example vitamins.

$$\frac{P}{\rho n k_b T} = 1 + r^2 b \rho n g\left(d^+\right) - (r-1)\left[g\left(d^+\right)-1\right] - \frac{r^2 a \rho n}{k_b T} \qquad (6)$$

- The Statistical Associating Fluid Theory (SAFT) Equation of State [11]: This equation is also especially suitable to describe complex molecules as well as strong interactions between these molecules, and it can be adapted to describe polymers. Few applications of this equation to systems with supercritical fluids have been described, as for example the correlation of solid-liquid-gas equilibrium data of mixtures of polymers with supercritical CO_2 [12].

- The Group Contribution (GC) Equation of State [13]: This equation allows the calculation of the interaction between molecules by a group contribution method derived from UNIFAC. Therefore, as long as the required group contribution parameters are available, this equation can be predictive because only pure component properties are required. Many applications of this equation to correlate both vapor-liquid and solubility data with supercritical fluids can be found in the literature [14, 15].

Rapid Expansion of Supercritical Solutions (RESS)

The Rapid Expansion of Supercritical Solutions (RESS) process is constituted by two main steps: In the first one, the supercritical fluid is saturated with the solute of interest with an extraction performed at high pressure, and in the second one, this supercritical solution is expanded to a lower pressure through a capillary nozzle or a similar device. Supersaturation is caused by the drastic reduction of the solubility during the depressurization, which is achieved by the mechanical process of the expansion through the nozzle. Therefore, the core aspect of mathematical models of this process is an accurate description of the expansion. This expansion can be divided into four consecutive steps, presented in Fig. 1: the inlet to the nozzle, the expansion through the capillary nozzle, and the formation of a free jet after the nozzle, which depending on the ratio between pre-expansion and post-expansion pressures can include a section with supersonic velocities ending on a Mach disc [16].

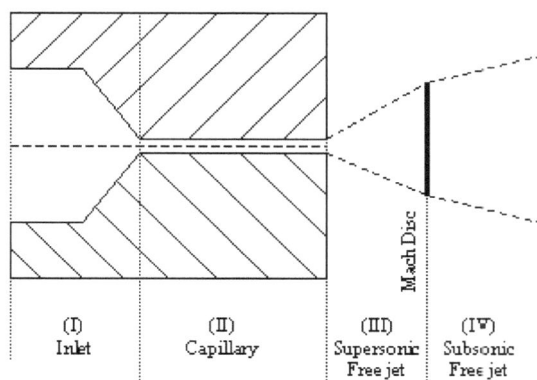

Figure 1: Consecutive steps in a RESS expansion device

A detailed mathematical model of the RESS process must consider the mass, energy and momentum conservation equations in the different sections of the expansion process. The most detailed models solve these conservation equations in the spatial coordinates [17], but as a simplifying assumption, a one-dimensional model can be considered, which considerably reduces the complexity of the calculations while maintaining a good accuracy. Helfgen *et al.* [16] presented a detailed description of the conservation equations required to model each section of the expansion, considering a one-dimensional model. Weber and Thies [18] presented a simplified model of the RESS process, with a discussion of the relative importance of the different aspects considered in the model.

A particularly complex aspect of the model is the description of the kinetics of particle formation and growth. Helfgen *et al.* [16] adapted a model originally developed for describing the evolution of liquid droplets in aerosols [19]. This model is based on a population balance to particles, which can be expressed through the General Dynamic Equation (GDE), presented in Eq. 7. This equation considers three different contributions: the formation of new particles by nucleation, the growth of particles by condensation, that is, by deposition of molecules of the solute over the particle, and the growth of particles by coagulation, which is related to the probability of two colliding particles to become stuck together forming a larger particle. To apply this equation, suitable models have to be used to calculate the rate of each of these contributions, and very frequently the main limitation of mathematical models is the lack of knowledge of the exact form of these rate equations, or of some of the physical properties required by them. Moreover, a rigorous resolution of the GDE involves the discretization of this equation over the entire range of possible particle sizes, which can be computationally demanding. Alternatively, a certain statistical distribution of particle sizes can be assumed (for instance, a Gaussian distribution), and then the GDE equation can be used to calculate the parameters of this distribution, according to the method of moments [16].

$$\nabla \cdot (\rho u N) = \underbrace{J(V^*)\delta(V - V^*)}_{nucleation} + \underbrace{\frac{1}{2}\int_0^V \beta(V - \overline{V}, V) \cdot N(V - \overline{V}) \cdot N(\overline{V}) \cdot d\overline{V}}_{coagulation} - \underbrace{N(V)\int_0^\infty \beta(V, \overline{V}) \cdot N(\overline{V}) \cdot d\overline{V}}_{coagulation} - \underbrace{\frac{\partial(G \cdot n)}{\partial V}}_{condensation} \qquad (7)$$

Model results regarding the fluid mechanics of the process [16] indicate that most of the pressure drop occurs in the supersonic free jet section. Pressure in this section of the jet can be below the bulk pressure in the expansion chamber; in this case, an increase in pressure is observed in the Mach disc. Depending on the conditions, the expansion path in the supersonic free jet can cross the phase boundaries, leading to the formation of liquid droplets of CO_2 or co-solvent, or even particles of solid CO_2. These phase transitions are frequently accompanied by drastic changes in the properties of the product, and it is normally advisable to avoid them [20]. Regarding the kinetics of particle formation and growth, most model results agree to indicate that the main mechanism of particle growth is coagulation during the expansion [16, 17, 18]. This theoretical result is in agreement with some experimental evidence that indicates a strong dependence of particle size with the design of the expansion chamber and of the particle collection system [21]. Weber and Thies [18] discussed the modeling of particle growth by coagulation under different conditions, and suggested several ways of limiting this growth in experiments, as for example reducing the time available for coagulation with an adequate design of the expansion chamber, using low concentration of particles as well as entrainment gases to reduce the probability of collisions between particles, or using surfactants to reduce the probability of coagulation when particles collide.

Particles from Gas Saturated Solutions (PGSS)

It is well known that one of the main limitations of the RESS process is its low production capacity, caused by the low solubility of most solutes of interest in the supercritical fluid. As the RESS process, the PGSS process consists in a saturation step performed at high pressure, followed by a depressurization in a nozzle. The innovation introduced with the PGSS process consists in expanding the CO_2-saturated liquid phase obtained in the extraction step, instead of the supercritical phase. Since the concentration of the solute in the liquid phase is much higher than in the supercritical phase, with this procedure the production capacity of the process is drastically increased. This change in the procedure also causes a variation of the driving force for the precipitation, which in the PGSS process is caused by the intense cooling effect due to the Joule-Thompson effect and the evaporation of CO_2 during the depressurization.

The saturation of the solute with the supercritical CO_2 also causes certain variations in its physical properties, which are positive for the performance of the process. When polymeric materials are PGSS-processed, the most notable changes in the physical properties of the polymer caused by CO_2 dissolution are a reduction of viscosity, a considerable swelling, and a reduction of melting and glass transition temperatures. The extent of the reduction of the melting temperature can be very high; of up to 30°C at moderate pressures [22]. As presented in Fig. **2**, the variation of melting temperature with CO_2 pressure is related to the solubility of CO_2 in the melt: at low pressures, melting temperature decreases almost linearly with pressure, and CO_2 solubility rapidly increases. At a certain pressure, CO_2 solubility reaches a "saturation" point, beyond which it is necessary to apply a very large increase in pressure to obtain a small increase in solubility. At this point, the melting temperature reaches its minimum value, and a further increase in pressure results in an increase of the melting temperature [23].

There are few references about the modeling of PGSS processes in the literature. However, it should be noticed that many features of the models of RESS processes can be adapted to describe the PGSS process. As it is the case with the RESS process, it is interesting to determine the Pressure-Temperature (P-T) trajectory followed by the fluid during the expansion. Since the beginning state of the solute in the PGSS process is a melted state, it is particularly interesting to establish if this trajectory will result in the solidification of the solute, or if it still will be a liquid, which is of course undesirable. Elvassore *et al.* [25] presented a thermodynamic model of the PGSS process that allowed obtaining the P-T expansion trajectory by solving the energy balance coupled with an Equation of State (Eq. 8).

$$\begin{cases} \Delta H = \left[x_{CO_2} H_{CO_2} + \left(1 - x_{CO_2}\right) H_{lip} \right] - H_{mix} = 0 \\ P = EoS\left(T, x_{CO_2}\right) \end{cases} \quad (8)$$

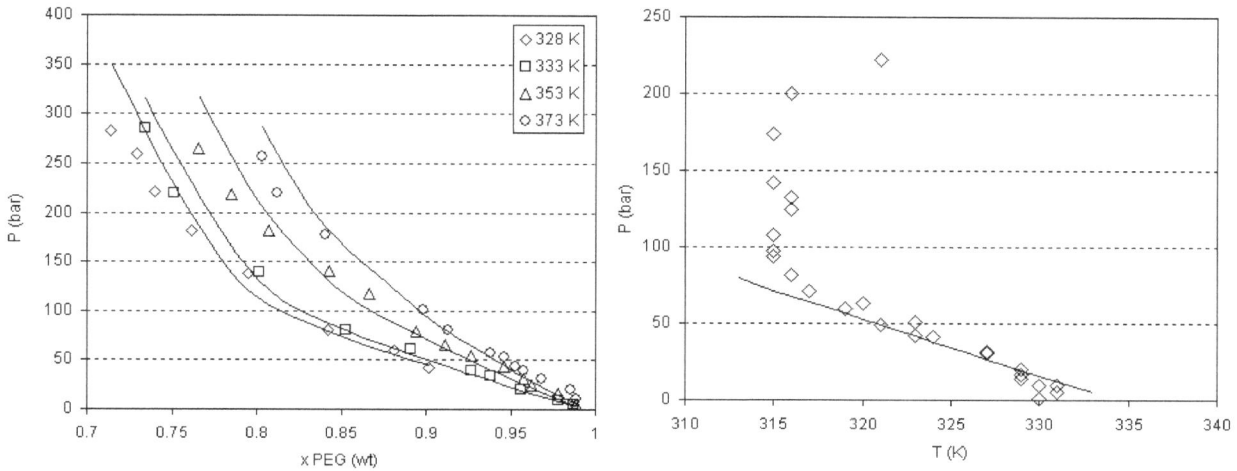

Figure 2: (a) VLE of PEG 4000 – CO$_2$ and (b) melting temperature of PEG 4000 under CO$_2$ pressure, experimental [23, 24] and calculated with the PHSC EoS

These authors used the Perturbed Hard Sphere Chain Equation of State to describe the thermodynamic properties of the system, and applied the model to study the precipitation of lipids. The model could be used to elaborate process charts, which specified the pre-expansion conditions that resulted in the formation of a solid, partially melted or liquid product.

Li *et al.* [26] presented a detailed model of the nozzle of the PGSS process. Their model was similar to the model of the RESS process presented by Helfgen *et al.* [16], and it considered mass, energy and momentum conservation equations, as well as particle formation and growth, described with the General Dynamic Equation for aerosols. The authors stated that a major difference between the PGSS and the RESS process is that, depending on the conditions, a two phase gas-liquid flow can take place inside the expansion nozzle, which can follow different flow patterns. Based on experimental observations, the authors postulated that the most likely flow pattern was dispersed bubble flow or drop flow for high flow rates, a type of flow pattern for which the two phases can be considered as a pseudo-phase, therefore enabling to describe the system with a one-dimensional, pseudo-homogeneous model. Model results indicated that since the residence time in the nozzle is extremely short, particles do not have time for growing by coagulation or condensation inside the nozzle. Since the authors did not include the free jet region in their calculations, model results underestimated experimental particle sizes by several orders of magnitude. It may be expected that, as in the RESS process, coagulation in the free jet is the main mechanism of particle growth in the PGSS process, and that therefore it is essential to include this region in the calculations in order to get accurate estimations of particle size.

Strumendo *et al.* [27] developed a model that described the evolution of one droplet of solution in the free jet region. The model considered the mass and energy transfer between the droplet and the surrounding gas. It allowed calculating the time required for solidification of the droplet, a piece of information which can be useful for calculating the size of the expansion chamber. However, the model included several simplifications and it did not consider the convective transport between gas and droplet.

Supercritical Anti Solvent (SAS) and related processes

At moderate pressures (10 – 15 MPa), supercritical carbon dioxide is very soluble or even completely miscible with many organic solvents. But at these pressures, the solubility of many solids of commercial interest in supercritical carbon dioxide is very low. The Supercritical Anti Solvent process exploits this property by using the supercritical fluid as an anti solvent that, upon mixing with a solution of the product in an organic solvent, causes its precipitation. An important advantage of this process over other anti solvent precipitation techniques are the good transport properties of the supercritical fluids, which allow a very fast and homogeneous saturations of the solution with the supercritical anti solvent.

Considering that the driving force for the precipitation with the SAS process is the anti solvent effect of sc-CO_2, and that the solvent power is strongly related to the density of the solvent, it has been found that the volumetric expansion of the organic solvent caused by the saturation of CO_2 is a very useful parameter for studying SAS precipitation processes. Two different definitions of the volumetric expansion have been proposed. The "classical" definition calculates the volumetric expansion as the ratio between the volume of the expanded solution and the initial volume, as presented in Eq. (9) [28]. De la Fuente *et al.* [29] proposed an alternative definition based on the analysis of the partial molar volumes, as presented in Eq. (10).

$$\frac{\Delta V}{V} = \frac{V(T,P) - V_0(T,P_0)}{V_0(T,P_0)} \qquad (9)$$

$$\frac{\Delta v}{v} = \frac{v(T,P) - v_0(T,P_0)}{v_0(T,P_0)} \qquad 10)$$

On a comparative study of the two definitions, de la Fuente *et al.* [30] showed that the "classical" definition (Eq. 9) does not distinguish the behavior of different organic solvents, while experimental results demonstrate that the results of the precipitation are different when different organic solvents are used. Moreover, the modified definition (Eq. 10) allowed the identification of suitable organic solvents for a certain application, and the selection of the optimum thermodynamic conditions for the precipitation: in the systems in which there is a sharp decrease in solubility at some concentration of CO_2, the performance of the GAS (Gas Anti Solvent) process will be adequate, since in this case the precipitation will take place very quickly and homogenously upon reaching this region. The systems which show slow decrease in solubility as the CO_2 amount increases are likely to yield worse results, since in this case the precipitation will take place continuously and relatively slowly as CO_2 is fed to the precipitator. These authors postulated that the optimum conditions for the GAS process are located in the minimum of the volumetric expansion curve of the solvent as defined by Eq. (10).

As it is schematically presented in Fig. **3**, depending on the position of the operating point with respect to the vapor-liquid diagram of the solvent-supercritical anti solvent system, two main regions of operation can be distinguished: above and below the mixture critical point. When the operating point lies below the mixture critical point, the supercritical solvent is partially miscible with the solution, and once that the solution is injected into the solvent, liquid jet break-up and atomization takes place, stabilized by the surface tension between the two fluid phases. However, when the operating point lies above the mixture critical point, supercritical fluid and solution are completely miscible and the equilibrium surface tension is equal to zero. Lengsfeld *et al.* [31] measured and calculated the jet break-up length. Their calculations included the variation of the surface tension with liquid and gas compositions. They concluded that the classic jet break-up theory could be applied successfully at subcritical conditions. However, at miscible conditions (above the critical point of the mixture organic solvent + CO_2), the surface tension decreases to zero in a shorter distance than characteristic break-up lengths. Therefore, distinct droplets are never formed at supercritical conditions, and the jet spreads forming a gaseous plume. In the intermediate region of near-critical conditions, the characteristic times of surface tension decrease and particle formation can be similar, and particles may be formed inside droplets of solution that disappear once the surface tension reaches equilibrium and vanishes to zero [32]. Experimentally it has been proved that the differences in the precipitation mechanisms in each of these regions lead to different product properties [33]. It must be taken into consideration that the presence of the solute may alter the phase boundaries. However, in many cases this influence is very small, and the phase diagram of the real ternary or multi-component system can be approximated by the binary phase diagram of the solvent – supercritical fluid system [34].

For operation at sub-critical or near-critical conditions, the surface tension between the solution and the supercritical fluid is a key physical property that determines the characteristics of the jet break-up and atomization processes. The surface tension can be calculated with the Parachor using Eq. (11), where the Parachor of each component can be calculated using a group contribution method [7].

$$\sigma^{1/4} = \sum_{i=1}^{n} [P_i](\rho_{Lm} x_i - \rho_{Vm} y_i) \qquad (11)$$

For the application of this method, it is necessary to know the density and composition of the phases in equilibrium. If this information is not known, it can be calculated with an equation of state.

If experimental information is available, the predictions with the Parachor method can be improved by modifying the exponent on the left side of Eq. (11). Typical exponents are in the range 1/3.4 to 1/4. Sun and Shekunov [35] used this procedure to fit the surface tension of the mixture ethanol-carbon dioxide. They found that the exponent of the equation that yielded the best fit were in the range from 1/3.3 to 1/4, depending on temperature.

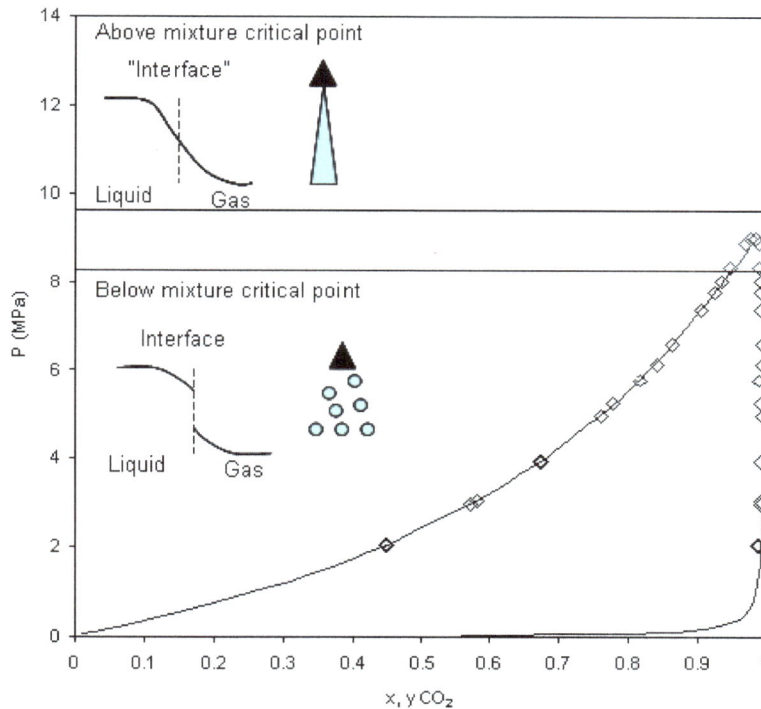

Figure 3: P-xy phase equilibrium diagram of CO_2 – ethyl acetate at 323 K, showing schematically the composition profiles at the interface and the liquid injection mechanisms in the regions above and below the mixture critical point.

A more fundamental approach for the calculation of the surface tension is the application of the gradient theory. With this theory, the interfacial tension is calculated as a function of the gradients of composition and density at the interface, which are calculated with an equation of state. Cornelisse *et al.* [36] used this method to calculate the interfacial tension in several binary and ternary systems. They concluded that the main factor that determines the accuracy of this method is the accuracy of the equation of state used for the density and composition calculations.

An aspect closely related to the surface tension, is the behavior of liquid jets injected into high pressure gases [37]. In this situation, it has been found that variations in pressure causes a modification in the atomization mechanism, due to the reduction in the surface tension, and to the increase in the drag friction found at higher gas densities. For this reason, with increasing pressure, a lower Reynolds number in the nozzle is required for achieving the atomization flow regime. Moreover, as previously described, the processes of jet break-up and atomization have also been observed at near-critical conditions or at conditions slightly above the mixture critical point. In this operation range, the formation of droplets and of a liquid jet is stabilized by the transient surface tension. Dukhin *et al.* [38] presented a detailed experimental and theoretical analysis of this situation.

Another important aspect in the operation at sub-critical conditions is the mass transfer between the liquid droplets and the surrounding gas. Werling and Debenedetti [39] developed a model that considered the two-way mass transfer of supercritical fluid and solvent between droplet and gas. The core equation of this model is the species mass balance, presented in Eq. (12). This model allowed to calculate the variation of droplet diameter with time, and in order to numerically solve the mass balances, a coordinate transformation was applied, as presented in Eq. (13). Some simplifications were included in the development of the model: only diffusive mass transfer was taken into account, considering that the gas phase was stagnant, and the system was supposed to be isothermal. As presented in Fig. **4**, model results indicate that droplet evaporation proceeds through two consecutive steps: in the first one, the droplet becomes saturated with CO_2, and droplet diameter considerably increases. This step is followed by the evaporation of solvent, a process that is comparatively slower than the first step.

$$\frac{\partial}{\partial t}(\rho x) + \nabla \cdot (-\rho D \nabla x + xN) = 0 \quad (12)$$

$$\xi = \frac{r}{R(t)} \quad (13)$$

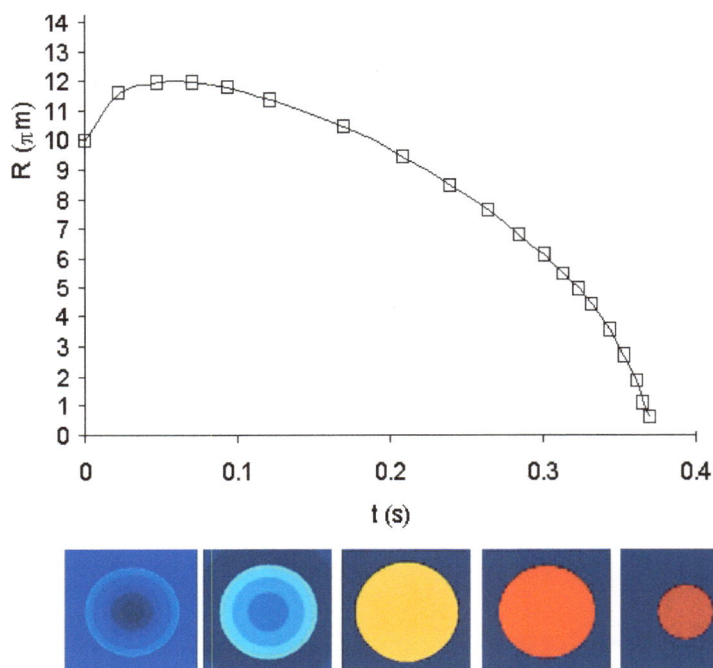

Figure 4: Evolution of droplet diameter during the precipitation of proteins from aqueous solutions [41]

Elvassore *et al.* [40] modified this model including the solute in the calculations, and Martín *et al.* [41] adapted this model to describe the precipitation of proteins from aqueous solutions, including the energy balance in the calculations. A different approach was followed by Pérez de Diego *et al.* [42], who took into account the convective mass transfer using adequate mass transfer coefficient correlations, and used a Maxwell-Stefan approach to calculate the multi-component mass transfer. Moreover, in contrast with the previous models, this model did not take into account the possible composition gradients inside the droplet. Nevertheless, model results showed the same qualitative behavior: a fast stage of droplet swelling caused by CO_2 solubilization, followed by a slower reduction of droplet size by evaporation.

With operating conditions above the mixture critical point, the plume formed by the injection of the solution into the supercritical fluid can be modeled using well-known computation fluid dynamic techniques. Martín and Cocero [43] developed a detailed mathematical model of the SAS process under conditions of total miscibility between supercritical fluid and organic solvent. The model included the mass and momentum conservation equations, which were solved numerically together with a k-ε model used to describe turbulence (Eqs. 14-18). The kinetics of particle formation and growth were described with the General Dynamic Equation for aerosols previously described (Eq. 7). This model allowed calculating the resulting particle size distributions. Model results were compared with experimental results obtained precipitating β-carotene by SAS. The calculated model results showed negative deviations with respect to experimental data, which were attributed to the lack of knowledge of some of the physical properties required to apply the GDE equation.

Continuity:

$$\frac{\partial}{\partial z}\left(\rho v_z\right)+\frac{1}{r}\frac{\partial}{\partial r}\left(r\rho v_r\right)=0 \qquad (14)$$

Species mass balance

$$\rho\left(v_r\frac{\partial \omega_a}{\partial r}+v_z\frac{\partial \omega_a}{\partial z}\right)=-\frac{1}{r}\frac{\partial}{\partial r}\left(rj_{ar}\right)+r_a \quad (15)$$

Momentum:

$$\rho\left(v_r\frac{\partial v_z}{\partial r}+v_z\frac{\partial v_z}{\partial z}\right)=-\left[\frac{1}{r}\frac{\partial}{\partial r}\left(r\left(\eta\frac{\partial v_z}{\partial r}\right)\right)\right]+\rho g \qquad (16)$$

Turbulent kinetic energy k and kinetic energy dissipation rate e

$$\frac{\partial}{\partial z}\left\{\overline{\overline{\rho k v_z}}\right\}+\frac{1}{r}\frac{\partial}{\partial r}r\left\{\overline{\overline{\rho k v_r}}-\left(\eta+\frac{\eta_t}{\sigma_k}\right)\frac{\partial}{\partial r}\overline{\overline{k}}\right\}=\overline{\overline{P}}_k-\overline{\overline{\rho\varepsilon}} \quad (17)$$

$$\frac{\partial}{\partial z}\left\{\overline{\overline{\rho\varepsilon v_z}}\right\}+\frac{1}{r}\frac{\partial}{\partial r}r\left\{\overline{\overline{\rho\varepsilon v_r}}-\left(\eta+\frac{\eta_t}{\sigma_\varepsilon}\right)\frac{\partial}{\partial r}\overline{\overline{\varepsilon}}\right\}=C_{\varepsilon 1}\frac{\overline{\overline{\varepsilon}}}{k}\overline{\overline{P}}_k-C_{s2}\frac{\overline{\overline{\rho\varepsilon}}^2}{k} \quad (18)$$

Henczka *et al.* [44] developed a Computational Fluid Dynamics (CFD) based model of the precipitation of paracetamol by the SEDS process. The model included the energy, mass and momentum conservation equations, using a k-ε turbulence model. The model allowed a quantitative prediction of the variation of particle size with the flow rates. M. A. Tavares Cardoso *et al.* [45] presented a CFD model that also took the effects of buoyancy and the excess volume of the mixture into consideration. This model allowed the identification of potential problems in the precipitation, as for example the presence of stratified regions inside the precipitator due to deficient mixing. Model results were also used to propose some practical hints for the optimization and scale-up of the precipitator, as for example the optimum design an location of CO_2 and solution injections, depending on whether the excess mixing volume is positive or negative.

CONCLUSIONS

Different approaches for the modeling of SCF precipitation processes have been presented. Solubility and other phase equilibrium calculations often are the most critical aspects of any model, because they provide the driving force for the precipitation processes. Cubic equations are suitable for correlation of experimental phase equilibrium data with simple substances, and other more physically realistic equations like PHSC, SAFT or GC-EoS are available when the phase behavior of complex systems (e.g. with polymers) has to be calculated.

Precipitation processes based on the use of supercritical fluids involve very complex phenomena. Mathematical models of these processes necessarily rely on simplifications and assumptions that allow focusing on specific aspects of the problem, neglecting others that are considered to be less important. In particular, the fluid dynamic aspects of the processes are not well known yet, and their influence on process performance is still open to debate. More fundamental studies of this aspect are required to fully understand the fluid dynamic mechanism of the process in order to be able to describe them with a rigorous model.

NOMENCLATURE

D : Diffusion coefficient (m^2/s)
f : Fugacity (Pa)
g : Gravity (m/s^2)
$g(d^+)$: Radial distribution function, PHSC EoS
G : Condensation rate (mol/m^3 s)
H : Enthalpy (J/mol)
J : Nucleation rate (mol/m^3 s)
k : Turbulent kinetic energy (m^2/s^2)
k_b : Boltzmann's constant (J/K)
n : Number of segments
P : Pressure (Pa)
P_i : Parachor of component i
P_k : Production of turbulent kinetic energy
$r.$: Segment radius (m)
R : Gas constant (J/mol K)
S : Supersaturation (-)
T : Temperature (K)
v : partial molar volume (m^3/mol); velocity (m/s)
V : molar volume (m^3/mol)
w : fluid composition (mass fraction)
x : Fluid composition (mol fraction)
y : Gas composition (mol fraction)
α : Parameter of Chrastil equation
β : Parameter of Chrastil equation
ε : Turbulent kinetic energy dissipation rate
η : Viscosity (Pa s)
ρ : density (mol/m^3)
σ : Interfacial tension (N/m)
ξ : Adimensional radial coordinate (-)

REFERENCES

[1] Martín, A.; Cocero, M. J., *Adv. Drug Delivery Rev.*, **2008**, 60, 339-350

[2] Brunner, G., Springer, Berlin, **1994**.

[3] Sauceau, J.-J. Letourneau, D. Richon, J. Fages., *Fluid Phase Eq.* **2003**, 208, 99-113.

[4] McHugh, M. A.; Watkins, J. J.; Doyle, P. T.; Krukonis, V. J., *Ind. Eng. Chem. Res.* **1988**, 27, 1025-1033.

[5] Kikic, I.; Lora, M.; Bertucco, A., *Ind. Eng. Chem. Res.* **1997**, 36, 5507-5515.

[6] Bertakis, E.; Lemonis, I.; Katsoufis, S.; Voutsas, E.; Dohrn, R.; Magoulas, K.; Tassios; D., *J. Supercrit. Fluids* **2007**, 41, 238-245.

[7] Poling, B.; J. Prausnitz, J.; O'Connell, J. P. The Properties of Gases and Liquids, 5th Ed. Mc Graw – Hill, **2001**.

[8] Constantinou, L.; Gani, R., *AIChE J.* **1994**, 40(10), 1697-1710.

[9] Song, Y.; Lambert, S. M.; Prausnitz, J. M., *Ind. Eng. Chem. Res.* **1994**, 33, 1047-1057.

[10] Colussi, S.; Elvassore, N.; Kikic, I., *J. Supercrit. Fluids* **2006**, 38, 18-26.

[11] Müller, E. A.; Gubbins, K. E., *Ind. Eng. Chem. Res.* **2001**, 40, 2193-2211.

[12] Wiesmet, V.; Weidner, E.; Behme, S.;Sadowski, G.; Arlt, W., *J. Supercrit. Fluids* **2000**, 17, 1-12.

[13] Skjold-Jorgensen, S., *Fluid Phase Eq.* **1984**, 16, 317-351.

[14] Espinosa, S.; Foco, G. M.; Bermúdez, A.; Fornari, T., *Fluid Phase Eq.* **2000**, 172, 129-143

[15] Espinosa, S.; Fornari, T.; Bottini, S. B.; Brignole, E. A., *J. Supercrit. Fluids* **2002**, 23, 91-102.

[16] Helfgen, B.; Türk, M.; Schaber, K., *J. Supercrit. Fluids*, **2003**, 26, 225-242.

[17] Franklin, R. K.; Edwards, J. R.; Chernyak, Y.; Gould, R. D.; Henon, F.; Carbonell, R. G., *Ind. Eng. Chem. Res.* **2001**, 40, 6127-6139

[18]   Weber, M.; Thies, M. C., *J. Supercrit. Fluids* **2007**, 40, 402-419.

[19]   Pratsinis, S. E., *J. Colloid Interf. Sci.*, **1988**, 124, 416.

[20]   Fagues, J. ; Lochard, H. ; Letourneau, J. J. ; Sauceau, M. ; Rodier, E., *Powder Technol.* **2004**, 141, 219-226

[21]   Subra, P.; Benoy, P.; Saurina, J.; Domingo, C., *J. Supercrit. Fluids* **2004**, 31, 313-322.

[22]   Tomasko, D. L.; Li, H.; Lui, D.; Han, X.; Wingert, M. J.; Lee, L. J.; Koelling, K. W., *Ind. Eng. Chem. Res.* **2003**, 42, 6431-6456.

[23]   Weidner, E.; Wiesmet, V.; Knez, Z.; Skerget, M., *J. Supercrit. Fluids* **1997**, 10, 139-147.

[24]   Wiesmet, V.; Weidner, E.; Behme, S.;Sadowski, G.; Arlt, W., *J. Supercrit. Fluids* **2000**, 17, 1-12

[25]   Elvassore, N.; Flaibani, M.; Bertucco, A.; Caliceti, P., *Ind. Eng. Chem. Res.* **2003**, 42, 5924-5930.

[26]   Li, J.; Matos, H. A.; Gomes de Azevedo, E., *J. Supercrit. Fluids* **2004**, 32, 275-286

[27]   Strumendo, M.; Bertucco, A.; Elvassore, N., *J. Supercrit. Fluids* **2007**, 41, 115-125.

[28]   Kordikowski, A.; Schenk, A. P.; Nielen, R. M. V.; Peters, C. J., *J. Supercrit. Fluids* **1995**, 8(3), 205-216

[29]   De la Fuente Badilla, J. C., Peters, J. C.; de Swaan Arons, J., *J. Supercrit. Fluids*, **2000**, 17, 13-23

[30]   De la Fuente, J. C. ; Shariati, A.; Peters, C. J., *J. Supercrit. Fluids* **2004**, 32, 55-61

[31]   Lengsfeld, C. S.; Delplanque, J. P.; Barocas, V. H.; Randolph, T. W., *J. Phys. Chem. B.,* **2000**, 104(12), 2725-2735.

[32]   Reverchon, E.; Adami, R.; Caputo, G.; de Marco, I., *J. Supercrit. Fluids* **2008**, 47(1), 70-84.

[33]   Reverchon, E.; de Marco, I.; Torino, E., *J. Supercrit. Fluids* **2007**, 43, 126-138.

[34]   Martín, A.; Gutiérrez, L.; Mattea, F.; Cocero, M. J., *Ind. Eng. Chem. Res.* **2007**, 46(5), 1552-1562.

[35]   Sun, Y.; Shekunov, B. Y., *J. Supercrit. Fluids*, **2003**, 27, 73-83.

[36]   Cornelisse, P. M. W.; Peters, C. J.; de Swaan Arons, J., *Fluid Phase Eq.*, **1993**, 82, 119-129

[37]   Czerwonatis, N.; Eggers, R., *Chem. Eng. Technol*, **2001**, 24, 619-624.

[38]   Dukhin, S. S.; Zhu, C.; Dave, R.; Pfeffer, R.; Luo, J. J.; Chávez, F.; Shen, Y., *Colloid Surface A* **2003**, 229, 181-199

[39]   Werling, J. O.; Debenedetti, P. G., *J. Supercrit. Fluids*, **1999**, 16, 167-181.

[40]   Elvassore, N.; Cozzi, F.; Bertucco, A., *Ind. Eng. Chem. Res.* **2004**, 43, 4935-4943.

[41]   Martín, A.; Bouchard, A.; Hofland, G. W.; Witkamp, G.-J.; Cocero, M. J., *J. Supercrit. Fluids* **2007**, 41(1), 126-137.

[42]   Pérez de Diego, Y.; Wubbolts, F. E.; Jansens, P. J., *J. Supercrit. Fluids*, **2006**, 37, 53-62.

[43]   Martín, A.; Cocero, M. J., *J. Supercrit. Fluids* **2004**, 32(1-3), 203-219

[44]   Henczka, M.; Baldyga, J.; Shekunov, B. Y., *Chem. Eng. Sci*, **2005**, 60, 2193-2201

[45]   Tavares Cardoso, M. A.; Cabral, J. M. S.; Palavra, A. M. F.; Geraldes, V., *J. Supercrit. Fluids* **2008**, 47, 247-258.

CHAPTER 6

Supercritical Fluid Impregnation for the Preparation of Controlled Delivery Systems

Ana Rita C. Duarte[1,2] and Catarina M. M. Duarte[3,4,*]

[1]3B's Research Group - Biomaterials, Biodegradables and Biomimetics, Dept. of Polymer Engineering, University of Minho, Headquarters of the European Institute of Excellence on Tissue Engineering and Regenerative Medicine, AvePark, Zona Industrial da Gandra, S. Cláudio do Barco, 4806-909 Caldas das Taipas, Guimarães, Portugal, http://www.3bs.uminho.pt; [2]IBB – Institute for Biotechnology and Bioengineering, PT Associated Laboratory (Laboratório Associado), Portugal, www.ibb.pt; [3]Instituto de Tecnologia Química e Biológica, Universidade Nova de Lisboa, Avenida da República, Estação Agronómica Nacional, 2780-157 Oeiras, Portugal and [4]Instituto de Biologia Experimental e Tecnológica, Avenida da República, Quinta-do-Marquês, Estação Agronómica Nacional, Apartado 12, 2781-901 Oeiras, Portugal; Email: cduarte@itqb.unl.pt

Abstract: Controlled drug delivery products, using biocompatible or biodegradable polymers, have received considerable attention in the last years. These substances provide in general a more controlled release rate of assumption of the drug by the body improving its therapeutic action. In fact, there is a growing interest of the pharmaceutical industry in the development of these systems. Impregnation using supercritical fluid technology has already proven its feasibility, in the preparation of controlled release systems. In this technique the drug component is dissolved in a compressed gas (carbon dioxide) that is used as a mobile phase and that, also, swells and stretches the polymer matrix, facilitating the diffusion of the drug, and increasing the rate of impregnation. A high purity product, free of residual solvents is obtained, since no organic solvents are involved in the impregnation process. In this chapter, the development of different successful controlled release systems is presented.

INTRODUCTION

Worldwide, there is an increasing concern on health care that creates a major opportunity for development of the new pharmaceutical formulations. Ageing populations worried about the quality of life in the older years are actively seeking for new, more effective and patient compliant drug delivery devices. This has been the driving force for the continuous growth of the research made on delivery devices, which has become a powerful technique in health care.

It has been recognized for long that simple pills or injections may not be the suitable methods of administration of a certain active compound. These medications present several problems and/or limitations, like poor drug bioavailability and systemic toxicity, derived essentially from pharmacokinetic and other carrier limitations and low solubility of the drugs in water. Therefore and to overcome these drawbacks, clinicians recommend frequent drug dosing, at high concentrations, in order to overcome poor drug bioavailability but causing a potential risk of systemic toxicity.

In many cases, conventional drug delivery products provide sharp increases in the drug concentration at potentially toxic levels, followed by a relatively short period at the therapeutic level and then drug concentration drops until new administration. In controlled drug delivery systems designed for long-term administration, the drug level in the blood follows the profile shown in Fig. **1**, remaining constant, between the desired maximum and minimum, for an extended period of time.

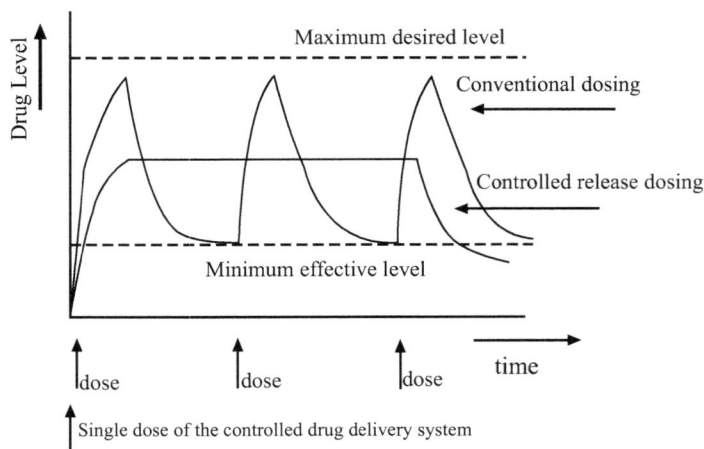

Figure 1: Drug concentration in blood after conventional dosing vs controlled release dosing

A controlled drug release system consists in a drug carrier capable of releasing the bioactive agent in a specific location at a specific rate [1].

Despite the number of advances made in the controlled release technology over the past two decades, the field is continuously growing.

The progress advances side by side with new drug discovery and new therapeutics, such as the research in gene therapy [2]. Furthermore, not only the drugs itself are being explored but also the technologies to prepare these new drug delivery systems. Major advances in the field of drug delivery and targeting have highlighted the limitations of the conventional particle formation and processing techniques [3, 4]. In the future, the intersection between nanotechnology and drug delivery may see exciting developments. [5]

Nanoparticulate technology is establishing its competence for several drugs and for an array of applications. The versatility, flexibility and adaptability of the nanoparticulate delivery systems have proven their potential to fulfill the need for improved health care and better patient compliance. The nanoparticulate delivery systems broadly comprise of polymeric nanoparticles, nanocapsules, solid lipid nanoparticles, and, recently, nanogels and drug nanoparticles have been included.

Pharmaceutical sciences are therefore experiencing a revolution as regards the existing technologies and the development of entirely new ones. Engineering drug itself in nanoparticulate form has emerged as a new strategy for drug delivery and supercritical fluid technology offers exciting opportunities in this field [6-10]. The application of supercritical fluids to the processing of pharmaceuticals has already proven its feasibility and also its applicability in the area of polymer processing [11-13] as well as in the preparation of controlled release systems [14, 15].

The pharmaceutical industry growing interest in controlled drug release systems coupled with the strict regulatory legislation are the driver forces to a world-wide intensive research in the supercritical fluid field. Particularly important issues for the pharmaceutical industry are to achieve a clean and environmentally friendly, single-step operation for the production of these systems. Supercritical fluids provide an attractive platform technology to meet the demands of the industry [3]. Nevertheless, any advantage has to be weighted against the cost and inconvenience of the higher pressures needed.

SCF technology comprises several processes, leading to very different particles in terms of size, shape, and morphology, that offer various possibilities to address the different issues to be solved and to prepare various forms or formulations of the drug: dry inhalable powder, nanoparticle suspension, microspheres or microcapsules of drug embedded in a carrier, drug impregnated excipient or matrix, etc. [9] The processes for the particle design using SCF can be classified in two main basic concepts: particle formation and impregnation [9, 17-19]. Particle formation or the precipitation of solids with dense gases presents several advantages over conventional processes of crystallization, such as fluid energy mill, spray drying, lyophilization, solution preparation and freeze-drying. The possibility of producing very small particles with a narrow size distribution using mild and inert conditions represents a major improvement over the conventional processes. Different particle formation processes based on supercritical fluids are available, including precipitation from supercritical solutions and precipitation using the supercritical fluid as non-solvent.

Supercritical Fluid Impregnation

Impregnation of a polymer matrix by a drug component dissolved in a supercritical fluid is a single component adsorption or absorption process governed by the solubility of the drug component in the supercritical fluid, the solubility of the SCF in the matrix (sorption and swelling determine the ease of impregnation) and the partition coefficient of the drug between the supercritical fluid and the polymer phases [15]. The impregnation process is then feasible, when the active substance is soluble in the supercritical fluid, the polymer swollen by the supercritical solution and the partition coefficient is favorable enough to allow the matrix to be charged with enough solute [14].

The use of a supercritical fluid for the preparation of polymer-drug formulations with molecularly dispersed drug molecules provides an alternative clean technology for conventional processes. This process can take advantage of the enhanced mass transfer provided by the use of supercritical fluid and the ease of solvent removal, which will result in a final product for human consumption completely free of any residual solvent contamination [10].

The application of supercritical fluid impregnation for pharmaceutical purposes has not been extensively studied in the past years, which is clearly evidenced by the few publications in this field. The studies reported in literature include:

-    impregnation of PVP with ibuprofen [20]

-    impregnation of PMMA/PCL blends with cholesterol [21]

-    impregnation of PLGA with 5-fluorouracil and b-estradiol [15]

-    impregnation of PVPPhys with ketoprofen, nimensulide and piroxicam [22]

-    impregnation of PMMA with hydroxybenzoic acid [23]

-    impregnation of P(MMA-EHA-EGDMA) with flurbiprofen [24]

-    impregnation of ethylcellulose/methylcellulose with naproxen [25]

-    impregnation of chitosan with indomethacin [26]

Supercritical fluid impregnation has also been applied for the preparation of controlled release systems from molecularly imprinted polymers. [27] Molecular imprinting is a new method to synthesise materials with sites of specific molecular arrangements that act as artificial receptors, on an otherwise uniform matrix [28].

The design of a precise macromolecular structure that is able to recognize specific molecules has indeed a large number of potential applications. There is a tremendous interest in analytical applications, such as biosensors, immunoassays, separation media and affinity supports among others [29]. Molecular imprinting has already given proofs of its enormous potential in the field of pharmaceutical applications [30]. In fact, in the last few years, the development of this technology has moved towards the preparation of new controlled release systems, where it may enhance the drug loading.

In this chapter supercritical fluid technology is described for the preparation of different controlled release systems. It was specially focused in supercritical fluid impregnation, as this process is still not completely explored for pharmaceutical applications. Few publications appear in this field although from the results obtained it seems very promising for the development of new controlled release systems.

EXPERIMENTAL

Supercritical fluid impregnation

A schematic representation of the process is presented in Fig. **2**. For the impregnation process of the polymer matrix, the SCF saturated with the drug component is passed over the polymer at a constant rate. During this process, it diffuses into the polymeric matrix, where the drug component is adsorbed on the polymer and entrapped as the systems is depressurized [14].

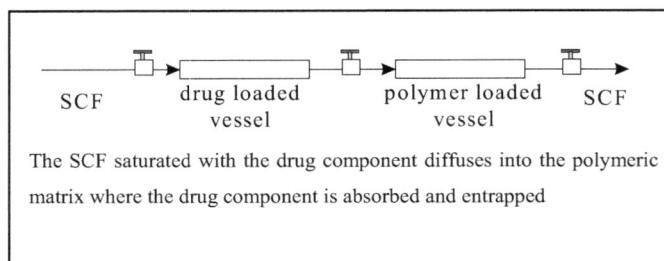

The SCF saturated with the drug component diffuses into the polymeric matrix where the drug component is absorbed and entrapped

Figure 2: Schematic representation of the SCF impregnation process

Supercritical Antisolvent Precipitation

In this process, the solute(s) are dissolved in an organic solvent, which is contacted with a supercritical solvent. The principle of this process is to decrease the solvent power of the liquid by addition of an anti-solvent in which the solute is insoluble.

A schematic representation of the process is presented in Fig. **3**. The formation of the particles is based on two mechanisms that take place simultaneously. On one hand, the solvent evaporates on the supercritical fluid and on the other hand the fluid penetrates into the droplets where it acts as an anti-solvent for the dissolved material so that precipitation occurs.

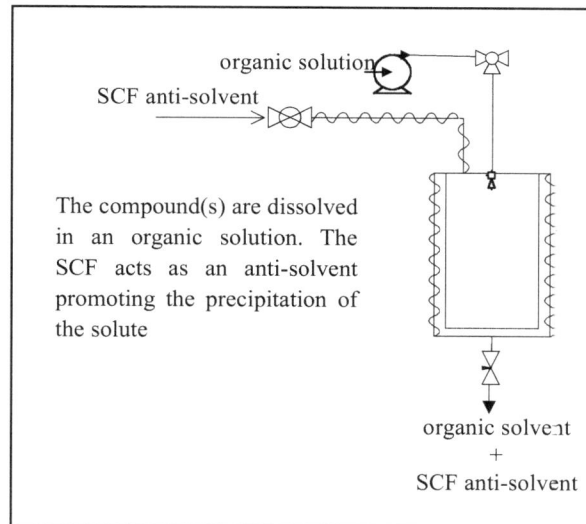

Figure 3: Schematic representation of the SAS process

RESULTS AND DISCUSSION

Controlled drug delivery systems can be prepared by the use of supercritical fluid technology and this chapter focuses mainly on the supercritical fluid impregnation process. The impregnation of polymeric materials was carried out, as polymers represent the most versatile class of materials. Furthermore, when a pharmaceutical compound is impregnated, encapsulated or attached to a carrier, such as a polymer, drug safety and efficacy can be greatly improved and new therapies are possible.

Different drug delivery systems were prepared using supercritical fluid impregnation.

Impregnation of polymeric films

Films of P(MMA-EHA-EGDMA) were impregnated with flurbiprofen for the preparation of a new ophthalmic drug delivery device and different operational conditions were tested in order to better understand the impregnation mechanism [24]. The polymeric films were analysed using scanning electron microscopy in order to evaluate the success of the impregnation. Fig. **4** presents a cross-section of a film impregnated with flurbiprofen.

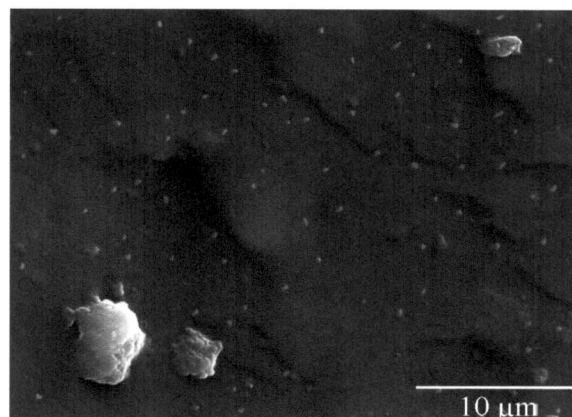

Figure 4: SEM image of a cross sectional cut of the film P(MMA-EHA-EGDMA) impregnated with flurbiprofen

Impregnation efficiency results from a complex mechanism that, in turn, involves interactions between the solute, the carrier and the matrix. The relative strength of all binary interactions will contribute to the final partitioning of the solute between the mobile phase and the solid. Flurbiprofen has a rather high solubility in carbon dioxide and it increases with pressure. Additionally, the sorption of carbon dioxide in the matrix also increases with pressure for a certain temperature. So it would be expected an increase of the solute uptake with pressure, on the basis that the more the CO_2 is loaded with the drug and the easier it goes inside the polymer, the larger should be the drug uptake. But, it is the contrary that is observed (Table **1**)

Table 1: Percentage of impregnation vs operational pressure

Experiment #	Pressure (MPa)	% impregnation
1	10.0	0.37
2	15.0	0.27
3	18.0	0.22

Indeed, the experiments show that these two effects when combined do not favour the impregnation process. This might be due to stronger interactions of the drug for the solvent (carbon dioxide) than for the polymeric matrix that is poorly impregnated.

Another revolutionary ophthalmic drug delivery device was developed based on commercially available soft contact lenses, which were impregnated with this same anti-inflammatory agent [31]. Cross-sections of the impregnated films were characterized using SEM imaging and two examples of a FOCUS DAILIES® lens impregnated with flurbiprofen are presented in Fig. **5**.

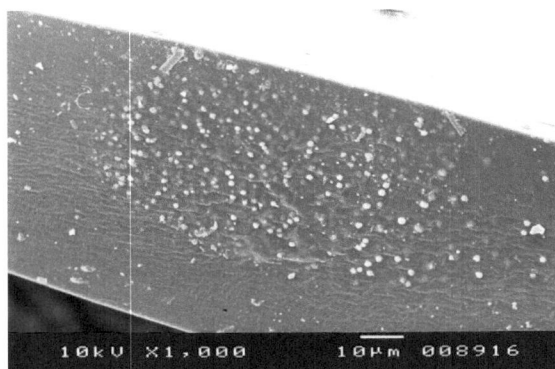

Figure 5: SEM image of a cross sectional cut of Focus® Dailies® lens impregnated with flurbiprofen

The release profiles of the samples prepared were performed in simulated lacrimal fluid. Fig. **6** illustrates the release profile in terms of drug concentration of a contact lens impregnated at 80.0 MPa and 313 K. As it can be observed the operating conditions have a great importance on the amount of drug impregnated in the polymeric matrix. A sustained release of flurbiprofen from the lenses was achieved up to eight hours.

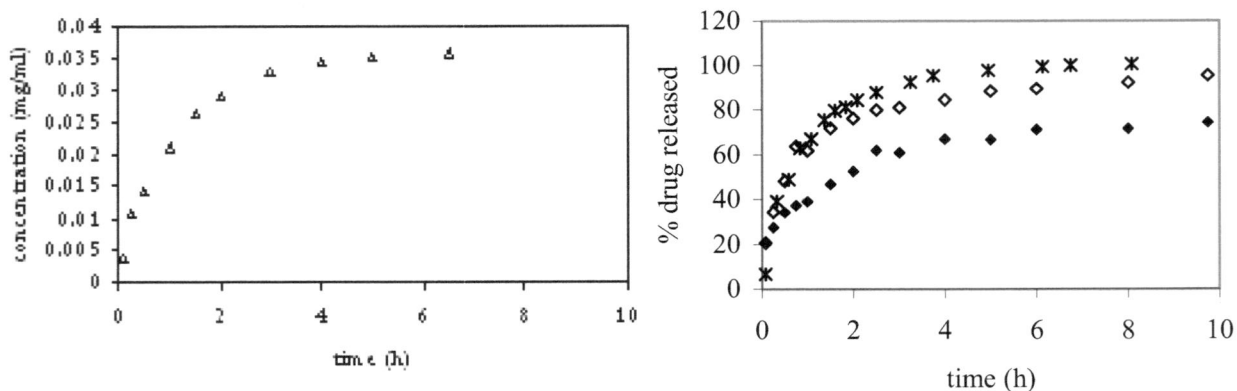

Figure 6: Release profile of flurbiprofen from the impregnated soft contact lenses

Impregnation of Polymeric Powders

The preparation of composite particles impregnated with an active compound can be achieved using two different techniques, either by supercritical fluid impregnation or by supercritical antisolvent precipitation (SAS)

Composite particles of acetazolamide + Eudragit were precipitated using the Supercritical Antisolvent (SAS) precipitation technique. [32] Different types of Eudragit polymers were used in order to prepare different composite particles with different drug release profiles.

Particles produced by the SAS process were recovered as a powder made of spherical and elongated structures, as shown in Fig. **7**.

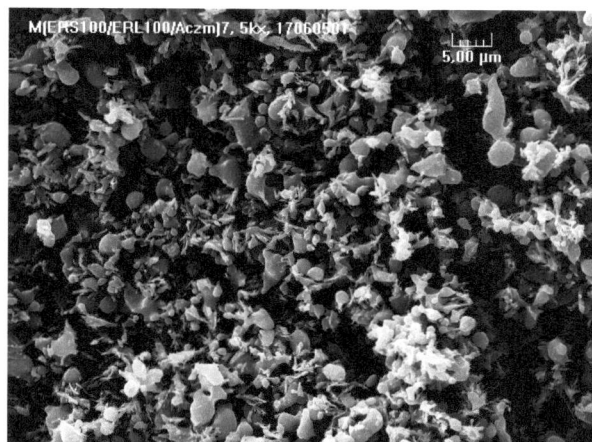

Figure 7: SEM image of the precipitated acetazolamide + Eudragit blend

The composition of the polymer mixture does not influence notably the yield or the mean particle size. However, it has a strong influence in the drug release profile (Fig. **8**) The release behaviour depends greatly on the type of polymer used in the formulation. Indeed, there is a large difference in the acetazolamide release from Eudragit RS 100 or from Eudragit RL 100, as illustrated in Fig. **8**.

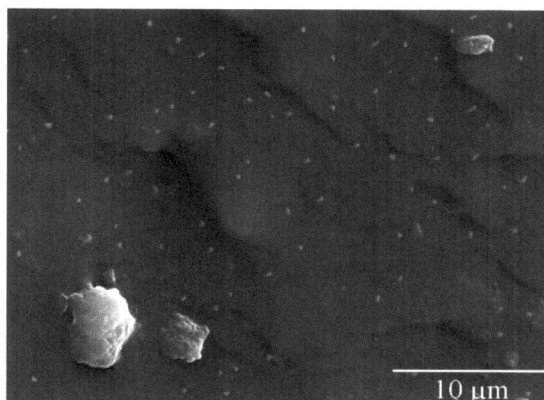

Figure 8: Release profiles of the (*) pure drug and the systems (t) Eudragit RS 100 + acetazolamide and (à) Eudragit RL 100 + acetazolamide

Acetazolamide release from Eudragit RS 100 miscrospheres was much slower and incomplete when compared to the spheres prepared with Eudragit RL 100 in which almost 80% of the drug is released after 3 hours.

Polymer powders of ethyl cellulose/methyl cellulose blends were also impregnated [25]. Ethyl cellulose is a widely used drug carrier and the extent of drug release from this matrix can be controlled by the addition of a water-soluble or water-swellable polymer, such as methylcellulose, which leads to the enhancement of poorly-water soluble molecules. Naproxen-loaded ethyl cellulose/methyl cellulose blends were prepared using different techniques.

The release profiles of the different systems prepared were performed. For the same polymeric blend is clear that the techniques used to both prepare and impregnate the microspheres influence the percentage of impregnated drug. Fig. **9** illustrates the release profile and it can be observed that the trends of the curves are different suggesting that they present different kinetics, therefore different release rates.

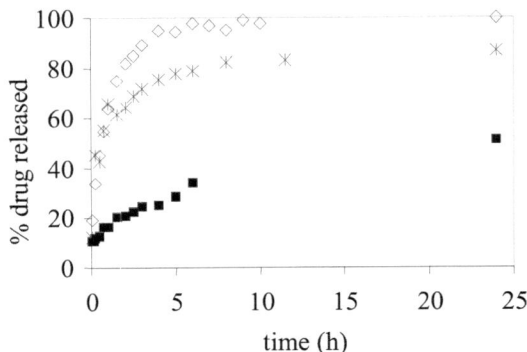

Figure 9: Release profiles of the systems prepared with 0.25 (%w/v) methylcellulose by (•) solv-evap + sc impregnation; (*) SAS + sc impregnation; (◊) solv-evap

The release rates are higher when the microspheres were prepared using the solvent-evaporation technique and lower in the case that particles were prepared by the conventional technique and impregnated with CO_2. Particles prepared by solvent-evaporation and impregnated using supercritical fluid technology present a very slow release profile, only 40% of the drug is released after 8-10 hours. Considering that these microspheres were prepared for oral medication and since the gastrointestinal transit time is considered to be 6-8 hours, as reported by Davis [33]

the particles prepared using solvent evaporation or supercritical fluid technology seem to be the most promising ones. From the results obtained it is possible to conclude that the size and shape of the particles impregnated has a great influence on the drug release profiles and therefore, tailor-made particles can be created using different combinations of particle production and impregnation techniques.

Molecularly Imprinted Polymers

A first attempt to prepare molecularly imprinted polymers using supercritical fluid technology a highly cross-linked polymer was prepared and acetylsalisylic acid was used as template molecule [27]. Poly(diethylene glycol dimethacrylate), PolyDEGDMA, was synthesised in supercritical carbon dioxide (scCO₂) in the presence of a template molecule of the active compound that was impregnated in the matrix in a subsequent step (Fig. **10**).

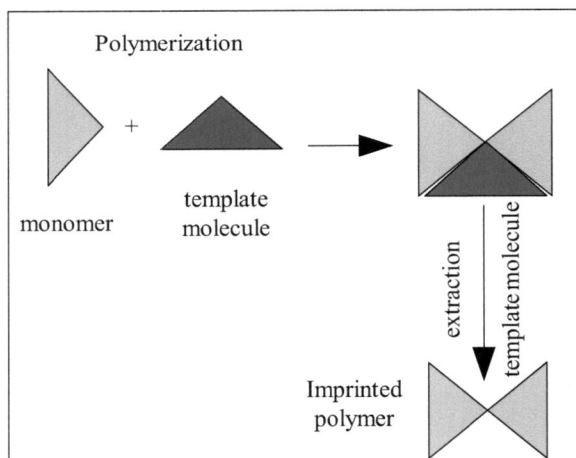

Figure 10: Scheme of the imprinting process.

Non-imprinted polyDEGDMA was successfully impregnated with acetylsalicylic acid, however, when the same polymer is polymerised in the presence of a residual amount of drug the concentration of impregnated drug is higher. Different percentages of the template were used in the polymerisation process in order to check the dependence of the degree of impregnation with the amount of drug present in the polymerisation. Acetylsalicylic acid was successfully impregnated in all cases, in fact, there is a correlation between the quantity of template present in the preparation of the MIPs and the percentage of impregnation. A higher concentration of the drug during the polymerisation step leads to higher percentages of impregnation (Fig. **11**). Acetylsalicylic acid-loaded

PolyDEGDMA miscrospheres were able to sustain drug release for several hours maintaining the drug concentration within eight hours.

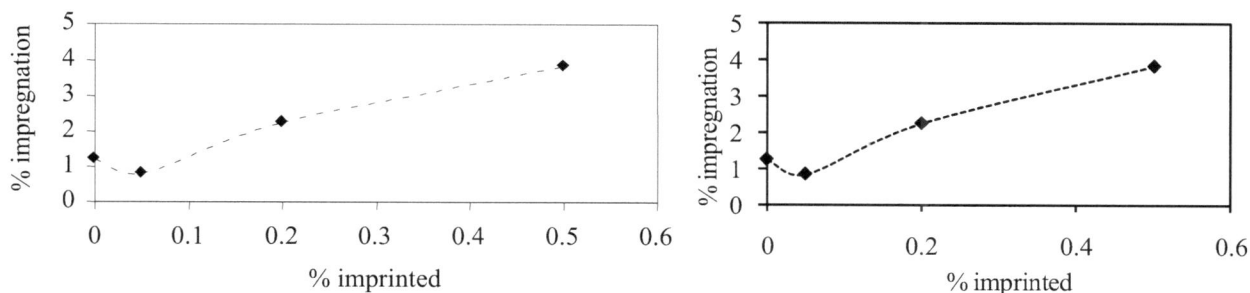

Figure 11: Percentage of impregnation of the systems PolyDEGDMA + acetylsalicylic acid as a function of the different percentages of template molecule present upon the imprinting process

CONCLUSIONS

In this chapter supercritical fluid technology was reviewd for the preparation for different controlled release systems. It was specially focused in supercritical fluid impregnation, as this process is still not completely explored for pharmaceutical applications. Few publications appear in this field although from the results obtained it seems very promising for the development of new controlled release systems.

Successful drug release systems were prepared with ophthalmic purposes, namely impregnation of a biocompatible polymeric film proposed for the preparation of intraocular lenses (of poly(methylmethacrylate-co-ethylhexylacrylate-coethyleneglicoldimethacrylate) P(MMA-EHA-EGDMA)) and commercially available contact lenses.

These matrixes were impregnated with flurbiprofen, an anti-inflammatory agent commonly used in the treatment of inflammatory diseases of the eye. This drug was used as a model drug and this impregnation process has the potential to be used with other pharmaceutical compounds for the treatment of more severe eye diseases, like glaucoma. The success of the impregnation depends greatly on the solubility of the drug in carbon dioxide and on the sorption of the fluid phase in the polymeric matrix.

Other drug release systems were prepared from polymer powders. Ethyl cellulose/methyl cellulose blends, prepared by two different methods (conventional solvent-evaporation and supercritical fluid anti-solvent technique) were impregnated with naproxen, another anti-inflammatory agent which solubility in carbon dioxide is described in literature. The supercritical anti-solvent (SAS) process presents enormous advantages for the preparation of the polymeric microparticles when comparing with conventional technique, as the particles prepared have a smaller size diameter and a narrower particle size distribution.

The process technique used to prepare the delivery system is clearly a factor that influences the percentage of drug impregnated in the polymer microspheres. The particles prepared by solvent evaporation and impregnated using supercritical fluid technology presented a slower release profile and only 40% of the drug was released after 8-10 hours. Microparticles prepared and impregnated using the same technique showed a controlled release profile and almost all the drug was released during what is considered to be the gastrointestinal transit time.

The SAS process was also used to prepare composite particles of acetazolamide and different Eudragit mixtures. The presence of different types or different polymer ratios of Eudragit in the particles lead to the preparation of delivery systems with different release profiles.

The rate of the release of the drug into aqueous media could be controlled to some extend by the preparation of these particles by varying the ratio of two types of Eudragit as polymer blend. Formulations enriched in Eudragit RS lead to a slower release of acetazolamide than those enriched in Eudragit RL.

The potential of supercritical fluid impregnation was also evaluated in the preparation of molecularly imprinted polymers for controlled drug delivery. In this first attempt to prepare MIPs using supercritical fluid technology a highly cross-linked polymer was prepared and acetylsalicylic acid was tested as template molecule with successful results. The release profiles of the systems studied show that there is a correlation between the amount of template present during the polymerisation step and the percentage of impregnation.

Controlled drug delivery devices are designed to improve the safety and efficacy of drug administration in the human body. The chapter specially focused on supercritical fluid impregnation, which represents a step forward in the preparation of delivery devices, using a clean and environmentally friendly technology. Different successful examples of polymers impregnated with various pharmaceutical compounds are presented and the fundamental studies required for a better optimisation of the processes are described.

Supercritical fluid impregnation has proven in several cases its feasibility for processing pharmaceutical compounds. The good performance of this technique, its easy scale up and the one-step process fulfil the requirements for the successful implementation of this process at industrial scale.

REFERENCES

[1] Malafaya, P. B., Silva, G. A., Baran, E. T., Reis, R. L., *Cur. Op. Solid State Mat. Sci.*, **2002**, 6, 283-295
[2] Langer, R., *Science*, **2001**, 293, 58
[3] York, P., *PSTT*, **1999**, 2, 430-440
[4] Ginty, P. J., Whitaker, M. J., Shakesheff, K. M., Howdle, S. M., *Nanotoday*, **2005**, 42-48
[5] Date, A. A., Patravale, V. B., *Cur Op Coll Inter Sci*, **2004**, 9, 222-235
[6] Kakumanu, V. K., Bansal, A. K., *Business Briefing: Labtech*, **2004**, 70-72
[7] Reverchon, E., Adami, R., *J. Supercrit. Fluids*, **2006**, 37(1), 1-22
[8] Foster, N., *et al.*, *Ind. Eng. Chem. Res.*, **2003**, 42, 6476-6493
[9] Jung, J., Perrut, M., *J. Supercrit. Fluids*, **2001**, 20, 179 – 219
[10] Kazarian, S. G., *Supercritical Fluid Technology for Drug Product Development*, Marcel Dekker, Inc., **2004**, 343
[11] Kazarian S.G., *Polymer Science, Ser C*, **2000**, 42, 78-101
[12] Cooper A.I., *J. Mater. Chem.*, **2000**, 10, 207-234
[13] Yeo, S.-D., Kiran, E., *J. Supercrit. Fluids*, **2004**, 34(3), 287-308
[14] Kikic, I., Vecchione, F., *Cur Op Solid State Mater Sci*, **2003**, 7, 399-405
[15] Guney, O., Akgerman, A., *AIChE Journal*, **2002**, 48 (4), 856-866
[16] Perrut, M., Clavier, J.-Y., *Ind. Eng. Chem. Res.* **2003**, 42, 6375-6383
[17] Perrut, M., Jung, J., Leboeuf, F., *Int. J. Pharm.*, **2005**, 288, 3-10
[18] Fages, J., *et al*, *Powder technology*, **2004**, 141, 219-226
[19] nez, Z., Weidner, E., *Cur Op Solid State Mater Sci*, **2003**, 7, 353–361
[20] Kazarian, S. G., Martirosyan, G. G., *Int. J. Pharm.*, **2002**, 232, 81-90
[21] Elvira, C., Fanovich, A., Fernández, M., Fraile, J., San Román, J., Domingo, C., *J. of Control Release*, **2004**, 99(2), 231-240
[22] Alessi, P., Cortesi, A., Kikic, I., Colombo, I., *Proceedings of the 5th Meeting on Supercritical Fluids*, vol 1, Nice, **1998**
[23] Diankov, S., Barth, D., Vega-Gonzalez, A., Pentchev, I. and Subra-Paternault, P., *J. Supercrit. Fluids*, **2007**, 41(1), 164-172
[24] Duarte, Ana Rita C., Simplicio, Ana Luisa, Vega-González, Arlette, Subra-Paternault, Pascale, Coimbra, Patrícia, Gil, M.H., Sousa, Herminio C. De, and Duarte, Catarina M.M., *J. Supercrit. Fluids*, **2007**, 42(3), 373-377
[25] Duarte, A. R. C., Costa, M. S., Simplício, A. L., Cardoso M. M., Duarte, C.M.M., *Int. J. Pharm.*, **2006**, 308(1-2), 168-174
[26] ong, K., Darr, J. A., Rehman, I. U. *Int. J. Pharm.*, **2006**, 315 (1-2) 102- 106
[27] Duarte, Ana Rita C., Casimiro, Teresa, Aguiar-Ricardo, Ana, Simplício, Ana Luísa, and Duarte, Catarina M.M., *J. Supercrit. Fluids*, **2006**, 39(1), 102-106
[28] Allender, C. J., Richardson, C., Woodhouse, B., Heard, C. M., Brain, K. R., *Int. J. Pharm.,* **2000**, 195, 39-43
[29] Hilt., J. Z, Byrne, M. E., *Adv. Drug Del. Rev.*, **2004**, 56, 1599-1620
[30] Lorenzo, C. A., Concheiro, A., "Molecularly imprinted polymers for drug delivery", *J. Chrom. B*, **2004**, 204, 231-245
[31] Sousa, H.C. de, Gil, M.H.M., Leite, E.O.B., Duarte, C.M.M., Duarte, A.R.C.,, "Methods for preparing sustained-release therapeutic ophthalmic articles using compressed fluids for impregnation of drugs", EP Patent EP1611877 A1
[32] Duarte, A. R. C., Roy, C., Vega-González, A., Duarte, C. M. M., Subra-Paternault, P., *Int.. J. Pharm.*, **2007**, 332 (1-2), 132-139
[33] Davis, S. S., *J. Control Release*, **1985**, 2, 27-38

CHAPTER 7

Ionic Liquids and Carbon Dioxide as Combined Solvents for Reactions and Separations: The Miscibility Switch

E. Kühne [1,2], G.J. Witkamp[1] and C.J. Peters [1,3,*]

[1]*Laboratory for Process Equipment, Delft University of Technology - Faculty of Mechanical, Maritime and Materials Engineering, The Netherlands;* [2]*Fluid Flow and Flow Assurance, Shell Global Solutions International B.V., The Netherlands and* [3]*The Petroleum Institute, Chemical Engineering Department, Abu Dhabi, United Arab Emirates; Email: cpeters@pi.ac.ae*

Abstract: Ionic liquids (ILs) and carbon dioxide (CO_2) are emerging as candidates to replace volatile organic solvents in synthesis and extraction processes. ILs are a relatively new class of substances composed only of ions and liquid at temperatures below 100°C. As a major attractive characteristic, they have negligble vapor pressure - reducing solvent loss by evaporation and environmental pollution. When used simultaneously with carbon dioxide for reactions and extractions, the process will be based on non-toxic, non-flammable solvents and will be applicable for a wide variety of compounds. It has been recently shown that carbon dioxide can be used to split phases in homogenous one-phase systems with ILs. This miscibility switch allows reactions to be carried out in one phase, and by simply changing CO_2 pressure, extractions can be carried out more efficiently under heterogeneous conditions. This chapter presents an overview on ionic liquids and carbon dioxide, together with an explanation on the phenomenon of miscibility switch.

IONIC LIQUIDS

Ionic liquids (ILs) are organic salts composed solely of ions, and by definition, their melting point is found at or below the convenient, arbitrary temperature of 100°C (373 K). Usually, cations are large organic molecules and anions, small inorganic ions. Due to their high degree of asymmetry, packing of the molecules in the crystal lattice is very difficult and therefore crystallization is prevented; this is one of the causes of the low melting point found for ionic liquids in comparison with other inorganic salts which have extremely high melting point (for instance, sodium chloride has a melting point of 801°C).

The number of cations and anions that can be selected for the design of an ionic liquid is enormous. Since anions and cations can be selected for a specific need, ionic liquids became known as "designer solvents". However, the task of choosing the best combination of cation and anion is very hard: as estimated by Earle and Seddon, there are at least one million types of binary ionic liquids [1] and 10^{18} ternary ionic liquids are potentially possible to be selected. For comparison, about 600 molecular solvents are in use today [2]. Some of the most studied cations and anions are shown in Fig. **1**.

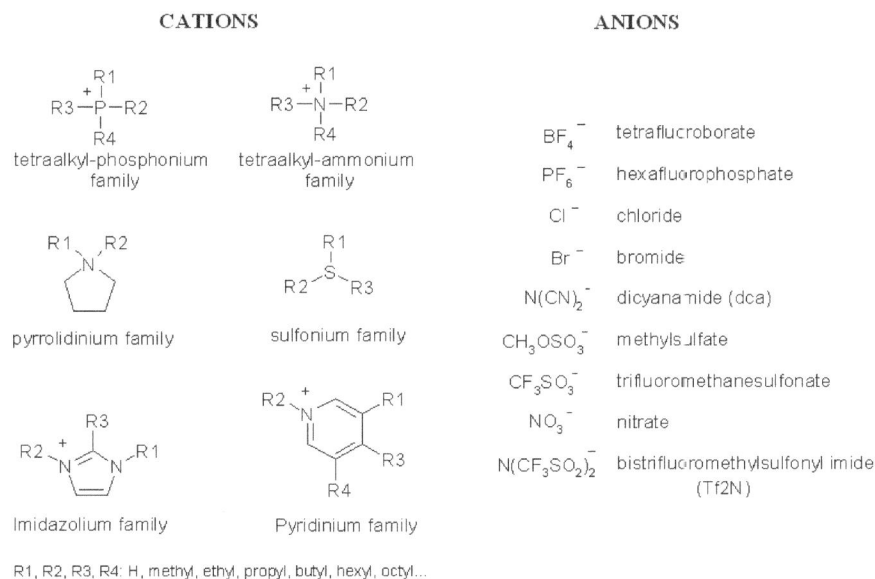

Figure 1: Some examples of the most popular anions and cations that can be selected for the design of an ionic liquid.

Ana Rita C. Duarte & Catarina M. M. Duarte (Eds)

Up to now, three different generations of ionic liquids are known. The 1st generation is comprised by chloroaluminate ionic liquids [3]. The 2nd generation is made of air and moisture stable ionic liquids [4], including bmim[BF$_4$]. Finally, the recently discovered task-specific ionic liquids belong to the 3rd generation [5, 6].

Ionic liquids called attention from industry and scientists due to some especial features, such as:

- They are known as "designer solvents" (they can be designed to have acid or basic characteristics, to be hydrophilic or hydrophobic, etc.);

- They have a large *liquidus* range of about 300°C (-96 to +200°C);

- Excellent solvents for organic, inorganic and polymeric materials;

- Negligible vapor pressure, detected only at extreme conditions of vacuum and at relatively high temperature [7, 8];

- Suitable density and viscosity;

- Thermally stable;

- Non-flammable;

- Wide electrochemical window;

- Nowadays commercially available and simple to synthesize.

However, ionic liquids are not intrinsically green, as they are commonly referred to. Toxic or flammable ionic liquids can be synthesized by the correct (or better said, wrong) combination of the cation and anion. Moreover, the synthesis of ionic liquids is also not performed at its best. It still resembles the traditional synthesis of most compounds, where litters of organic solvents are used and by-products are obtained. The development of more sustainable processes for synthesizing ionic liquids is necessary to completely evaluate the greenness of their use. In that respect, significant improvements have been done by synthesizing ionic liquids from renewable sources [9], by solvent-free anion exchange [10] and in supercritical CO_2 media [11]. Also biodegradable ionic liquids were recently synthesized [12].

One of the key features of ionic liquids is that physical-chemical properties can be tailored by a suitable combination of cations and anions. The major problem is that "the perfect" ionic liquid may not exist; with the improvement of some properties, other ones may be compromised. The effects of the different types of cations and anions on the final properties of the ionic liquids are presented in the next Section.

Properties of Ionic Liquids

Most of the intrinsic properties of ionic liquids derive from the Coulombic attraction forces between the ions. They determine not only the vanishingly low vapour pressure that is characteristic of ionic liquids, but for instance, also the melting point temperature. However, other effects such as van der Waals and hydrogen bond interactions and rotation of the alkyl chain length of the cation also influences the properties of ionic liquids. They are all closely related with the combination of cations and anions.

Computation of the melting point of ionic liquids is problematic, since glass transitions are sometimes wrongly reported as melting points [13]. Usually, an increase in the alkyl chain length of the cation from methyl to butyl or hexyl is responsible for a decrease on the melting point, and further increase results in aproportional increase of the melting point, since the asymmetry of the system also increases.

Water solubility, for instance, is strongly influenced by the anion. Considering the same cation, water miscibility increases in the following order: PF_6^-, $[(CF_3SO_2)_2N]^-$ < BF_4^-, $CF_3SO_3^-$ < $CH_3CO_2^-$, $CF_3CO_2^-$, NO_3^-, Br^-, Cl^- [14].

The viscosity of ionic liquids is still a problem to be overcome. It is several times higher than water and the most common VOC's, being comparable to some oils. This is a considerable disadvantage when mass and heat transfers are considered, as well as chemical processing (for instance, pumping and mixing). However, ionic liquids based on the dicyanamide anion ($N(CN)_2^-$) are very low viscous compounds, with viscosity at 20°C in the order of 21 cP (emimdca) up to 50 cP (N-butyl-N-methylpyrrolidinium dca) [15]. For comparison the viscosity of water at the same temperature is 1.002 cP, and the one of bmim[PF$_6$] is 430 cP [13].

The solvation and solubility characteristics of ionic liquids are also dependant on cations and anions [16]. A good example of anion influence in the solubility of a certain compound in ionic liquids is water miscibility. While some ionic liquids are extremely hygroscopic and therefore water miscible (for instance, IL's with the NO_3^- anion), other ones present miscibility gaps. When organic solvents are considered, the statement "like dissolves like" can not be applied. Many ionic liquids are miscible with organic solvents after their dielectric constant exceeds a certain value which seems to be specific for each cation and anion combination [16].

A summary of the influence of anion, cation and chain length in the properties of ILs can be seen in Table **1**.

Toxicity of Ionic Liquids

The toxicity of ionic liquids is still an issue when industrial application is concerned. Since the re-discovery of ionic liquids about two decades ago, researches were focused on finding new applications and collecting physical properties rather than understanding the risks that the use of ionic liquids may present to human health and environment. Fortunately, the last years have seen major improvements on the evaluation of toxicity, mutagenicity and environmental fate of ionic liquids. Due to its significance, a brief overview on these findings is presented herein.

The first attempts to investigate the hazards of ionic liquids have been made by the group of Prof. Bernd Jastorff, from the University of Bremen [19]. In his extensive program on ionic liquids toxicity, he focused on the effect of ionic liquid structure on eco-(toxicological) aspects. Their first results investigating different organisms showed that, disregarding the cation type, shorter alkyl chain length resulted systematically in a decrease of cytotoxicity [20].

These results were also confirmed by Docherty and Kulpa [21], who found that an increase in alkyl chain length as well as an increase in the number of alkyl groups substituted on the cation ring resulted in an increase in toxicity. However, in this study anion variation did not correspond to relatively different toxicities, in contradiction with a more detailed study from Jastorff *et al.* [20] and Stolte *et al.* [22]. Stolte and co-workers also discovered that lipophilicity and vulnerability to hydrolytic cleavage are keys for understanding and evaluating anion toxicity.

For comparison, Table **2** presents the values of the acute toxicity (LC 50, Lethal Concentration) to *Daphnia Magna* for ionic liquids and common chemicals used in industry [23, 24]. The lower the value of LC50, the more toxic the substance is considered. Above 10 mg/L, the substance is considered environmentally benign [25].

Table 1: Summary of some properties of ionic liquids and their dependence on the choices of cations and anions. [17, 18].

Property	Cation	Anion
Melting point	Decreases with increasing size of the cation and decreasing symmetry	Decreases with increasing size of the anion
Water solubility	Hydrophobicity increases with increasing alkyl chain length	Strongly affected by the anion type.
Polarity	Strongly affected by the cation type.	Less influenced by the anion choice
Viscosity	Increases with increasing cation size	Affects with no defined pattern.
Density	Decreases with increasing cation size	Affects with no defined pattern.
Conductivity	Increasing alkyl chain length decreases the conductivity	
Diffusion Coefficient	Increasing alkyl chain length decreases the cation diffusion coefficient.	Slightly increases with increasing anion size
Gases solubility	Little influence	Strongly affected by the anion type.

From the toxicity values of most imidazolium ionic liquids as presented in Table **2**, they can be considered environmentally friendly. A more detailed study based on a screening of different degrees of aquatic, terrestrial and cellular toxicity (genotoxicity, eye corrosivity alert, acute ecotoxicological alert and acute systemic toxicity alert) has been performed by Merck KGaA in collaboration with the UFT university in Bremen, Germany. A wide variety of ionic liquids have been studied, and as general conclusions, their results indicated certain (eco)toxicological concerns. Workers were advised to wear safety glasses when handling ionic liquids, since there is a risk of serious damage to eyes (results of HET-CAM testing). Potential for skin irritation cannot be excluded, and based on results of ecotoxicological screening, ionic liquids should be subjected to adequate waste disposal [26].

Regarding mutagenicity, Docherty and co-workers studied different ionic liquids and concluded that none of the imidazolium, pyridinium or quaternary ammonium ionic liquids can cause mutations [27]. However, they advise further experiments and deeper investigation on the subject before determining the carcinogenic potential of ionic liquids.

These efforts of industry and university are very encouraging, providing reliable information for the smart design of new ionic liquids. In summary, ionic liquids should not be generalized as "environmentally benign". To reduce toxicity, long side chains should be avoided in the design of cation structure, and a careful selection of the anion can lead to a less toxic ionic liquid.

SUPERCRITICAL FLUIDS

Supercritical fluids (SCF) are defined as any substance at a temperature and pressure above its thermodynamic critical point and which has a density close to or higher than its critical density [28]. The region where a supercritical fluid is found can be seen in Fig. **2**.

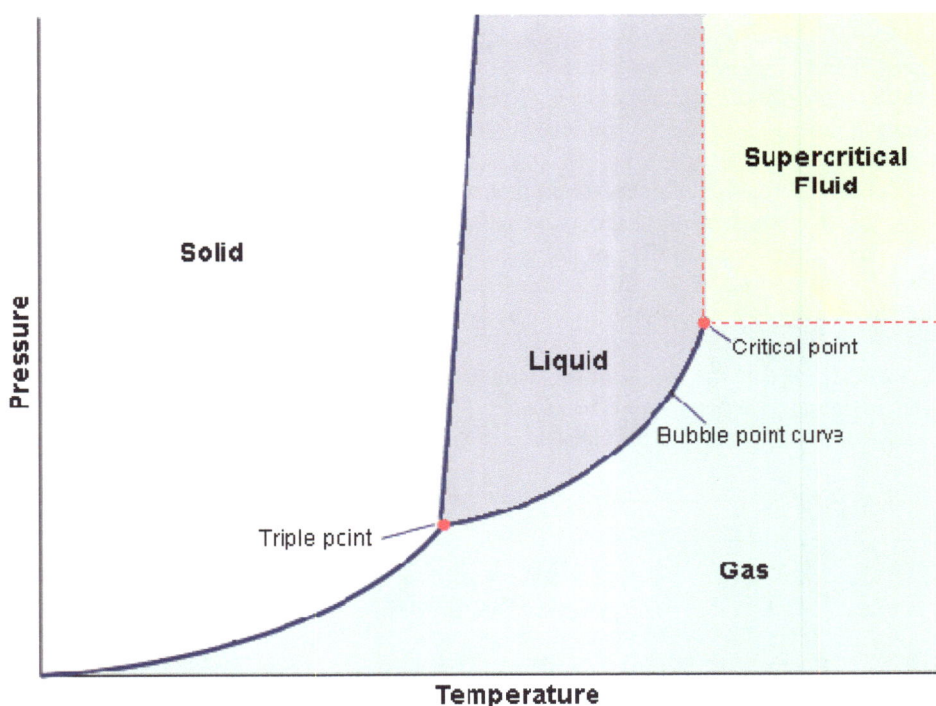

Figure 2: Location of the supercritical region in the phase diagram of a hypothetical pure compound.

The gas-liquid coexistence curve is known as the bubble point curve. By moving upwards along the bubble point curve, simultaneously increasing temperature and pressure, the liquid phase becomes less dense due to thermal expansion and the gas phase becomes denser as the pressure rises. Eventually, the densities of the two phases converge and become identical, making the distinction between gas and liquid not possible, ending the bubble point curve at the critical point.

Supercritical fluids possess properties of both gases and liquids, what makes them very attractive for material processing. For instance, the diffusivity in SCF is higher than the one in liquids, but viscosity is lower, facilitating mass transport. Because of the high compressibility, density and dissolving power can be tuned sensitively through small changes in pressure. Because of their tunable properties, supercritical fluids can be used in various applications with different nature of compounds. For more information on properties of SCF, the reader is referred elsewhere [29, 30].

However, the critical point of most compounds is found at extremely high pressure (P_c) and/or temperature (T_c) conditions, as shown in Table **3**.

Table 2: Acute toxicity of some compounds to *Daphnia Magna* (48h) [ξ] (based on LC50 values in mmol/L).

Substance	LC50 (mg/L)	Ionic Liquid	log LC50[ξ]
Chlorine	0.12-0.15	omim[Br]	-4.33
Ammonia (NH3)	2.9-6.93	1-*n*-Hexylpyridium Br	-1.93
Imidazolium ionic liquids	8.03-19.91	Tetrabutylammonium Br	-2.05
Phenol	10-17	Tetrabutylphosphonium Br	-1.53
Trichloromethane	29	bmim[BF$_4$]	-1.32
Tetrachlorometahne	35	bmim[PF$_6$]	-1.15
Methanol	3289	bmim[Br]	-1.43
Acetonitrile	3600	bmim[Cl]	-1.07

Table 3: Critical properties of diverse solvents [29].

Solvent	T$_c$ (^{o}C)	P$_c$(bar)
CO$_2$	31.1	73.8
Ethane	32.2	48.8
Ethylene	9.3	50.4
Cyclohexane	280.3	40.7
Toluene	318.6	41.1
Benzene	289.0	48.9
Water	374.2	220.5

Due to, among others, its low critical pressure and temperature, carbon dioxide has been the most studied supercritical fluid.

Supercritical Carbon Dioxide

Supercritical fluids are also good candidates for replacing VOS's. Among the most studied supercritical fluids is carbon dioxide: it is cheap, easily available, non-flammable, non-toxic and as it has seen in the previous section, has mild critical pressure and temperature. Carbon dioxide is relatively inert towards reactive compounds, but its relative inertness should not be confused with <u>complete</u> inertness. Carbon dioxide will react with strong bases (amines, phosphines, alkyl anions). When attempting to use amines as reactants this can be a serious disadvantage, in that carbamate formation can slow the rate of the intended reaction and can also alter the solubility characteristics of the substrate [31].

In the gas phase, carbon dioxide is volatile, non-viscous, no conducting, no polar, and unable to dissolve large and unsaturated compounds. When used under supercritical conditions, however, the solubility of organic compounds in CO$_2$ improves considerably.

The range of application for carbon dioxide is very large; it has been used for precipitation of drugs (for instance in the GAS process [32]), for extraction of natural compounds, as solvent for performance of diverse sorts of reactions, for processing of polymers, pharmaceuticals and waste streams, and various others [29, 31].

The combination of ionic liquids (polar solvents) and carbon dioxide (non-polar[1] solvent) generates a very flexible system applicable to a large number of compounds, both polar and non-polar. The advantages of this combination are presented in the next Section.

IONIC LIQUIDS – CARBON DIOXIDE SYSTEMS

The simultaneous use of ionic liquids and carbon dioxide in industrial applications is very interesting, especially because of their contrasting (and complementing) properties.

---

[1] The quadrupole moment of CO$_2$ is not considered in the affirmation that CO$_2$ is non-polar, but rather its low dielectric constant.

Against the statement "like dissolves like", ionic liquids can be considered good solvents for carbon dioxide. The extent of dissolution is dictated mainly by the anion type and its interactions with CO_2 molecules [33]. When CO_2 dissolves in the ionic liquid, negligible expansion of the liquid phase is detected [34, 35]. The strong interactions that keep the molecules of the ionic liquid close inhibit expansion when CO_2 is dissolved, increasing the density of the mixture. Although the molar volume expansion is small in comparison with common organic solvents, upon dissolution of CO_2 in the ionic liquid viscosity reduction and increase in hydrogen solubility also occurs [36, 14].

The interest in combining ionic liquids and CO_2 emerged from the difficulty of product separation when ionic liquids are used as solvents in, for instance, reactions. Since ionic liquids have extremely low vapor pressures, well-known processes like distillation are not an option, especially if the product is thermally unstable. The use of organic solvents for extraction is preferably avoided, since it compromises the green nature of the process. The challenge of separating compounds from ionic liquids can be overcome by extraction with supercritical CO_2, considered also a green solvent, as demonstrated by Blanchard and Brennecke [37]. One must be aware, however, that the main advantage of using ionic liquids in combination with $scCO_2$ for extractions (it means, negligible solubility of ionic liquids in the supercritical phase) can be influenced by dissolved polar compounds which may act as cosolvents, increasing the solubility of ionic liquid in the supercritical phase [38, 39]. Thus, previous studies about solubility of the involved components and ionic liquid in sc CO_2 are always necessary for extraction processes, including the effects of the interaction of those components in the system.

Another advantage arises from the use of CO_2 in combination with ionic liquid-organic mixtures. Previous research performed by Peters and Gauter [40, 41] showed that mixtures of the type liquid$_1$ + liquid$_2$ + CO_2 present miscibility windows, i.e., changes in carbon dioxide pressure are able to tune the miscibility of the phases. This phenomenon has proven to hold also for mixtures ionic liquid + organic + CO_2 [42] as well as ionic liquid + water + CO_2 [43], in which it has been demonstrated that carbon dioxide is able to induce phase separations also in systems with ionic liquids.

When ionic liquids and CO_2 are combined for reactions and separations, the switch in miscibility caused by changes in pressure can be used to the advantage of the process: reactions can be performed in a homogeneous system, and by pressure changes, separation of the reaction mixture into two or more phases (usually one organic–rich and one ionic liquid-rich) is possible, leading to high reactions rates, reduced mass transfer barriers and a more efficient separation of the product. Since ionic liquids have negligible solubility in CO_2 [34], the product can be extracted by the supercritical phase without any contamination from the solvents, achieving high purity levels of the final product.

Combining ionic liquids and carbon dioxide in reaction and extraction media has proved to be very attractive. Among others, the following advantages can be mentioned: both are non-toxic, non-flammable, carbon dioxide is cheap and has mild critical properties, and ionic liquids are nowadays available commercially at reasonable prices. Moreover, the switch in miscibility to perform reactions in one homogeneous phase and further extraction in a two-phase system offers higher reaction rates, a more efficient extraction and easy separation of the product, since no traces of ionic liquid will be found in the supercritical phase [42]. Therefore, products can be obtained with high purity, recycling of both solvents is possible and since the catalyst can be immobilized in the ionic liquid phase [44], no catalyst leaching will occur. An example of a process in which carbon dioxide is used to tune the miscibility of the system as well as to extract the product from the reaction mixture has been designed by Kroon and co-workers [45] and is schematically represented in Fig. **3**.

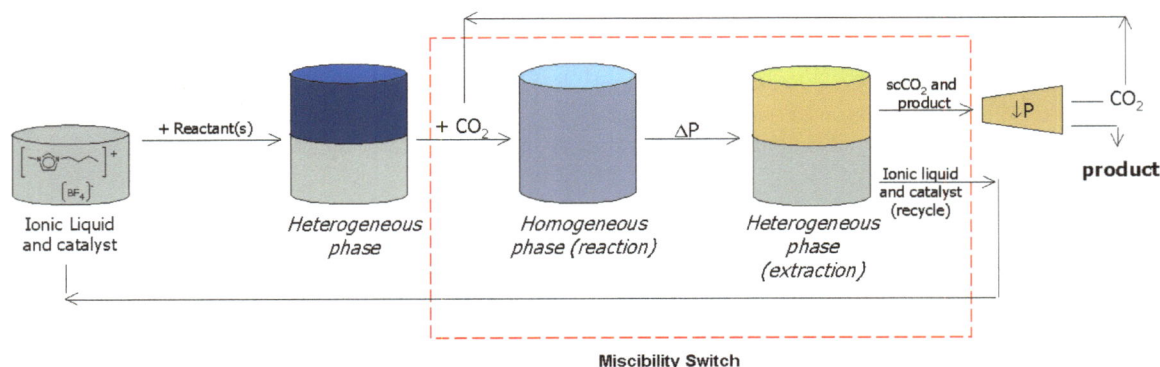

Figure 3: Simplified scheme of a green synthesis and extraction process in an ionic liquid-CO_2 medium. The red-dashed box indicates the part of the process where the miscibility switch plays an important role, and where knowledge of the phase behavior of the system is of fundamental importance.

THE MISCIBILITY SWITCH

The first set of phase diagrams describing the effect of carbon dioxide on the miscibility switch phenomenon in systems with ionic liquids have been presented by Florusse *et al.* [46]. From an investigation of the phase behaviour of the system CO_2 + 1-hexyl-3-methylimidazolium tetrafluoroborate + isopropanol they discovered that, for a constant ratio ionic liquid : isopropanol, an increase in CO_2 composition from 52 mol% until 60 mol% shifted the location of the homogeneous liquid region upwards in pressure, and decreased its size at constant pressure, until complete disappearance occurred.

This phenomenon is shown in Fig. **4**. From this figure the effect of carbon dioxide in the miscibility of the system is very clear. The progress of the two L_1+L_2 phase boundaries approaching each other and reducing the extension of the homogeneous liquid region is easily seen is diagrams A and B, while in diagram C the L+V phase boundary gives place to a very narrow three-phase L_1+L_2+V region.

The small range of carbon dioxide composition in which this phenomenon is found justifies why it is sometimes easily missed during phase behavior measurements. Although it has been assumed to occur with any ternary system of the type liquid$_1$ + liquid$_2$ + CO_2 [40, 41] and to be easily predicted from simple equations of state [47] the complexity of mixtures with ionic liquids makes the identification of the miscibility switch phenomenon a challenge. In principle, the location of the homogeneous liquid region is unknown, and so is the range of carbon dioxide composition under which the behavior as presented in Fig. **4** is comprised. In that respect, the nature of the interactions between the components of the ternary mixture plays an important role in defining the location of the phase boundaries of the system and therefore, the complexity of the miscibility switch identification.

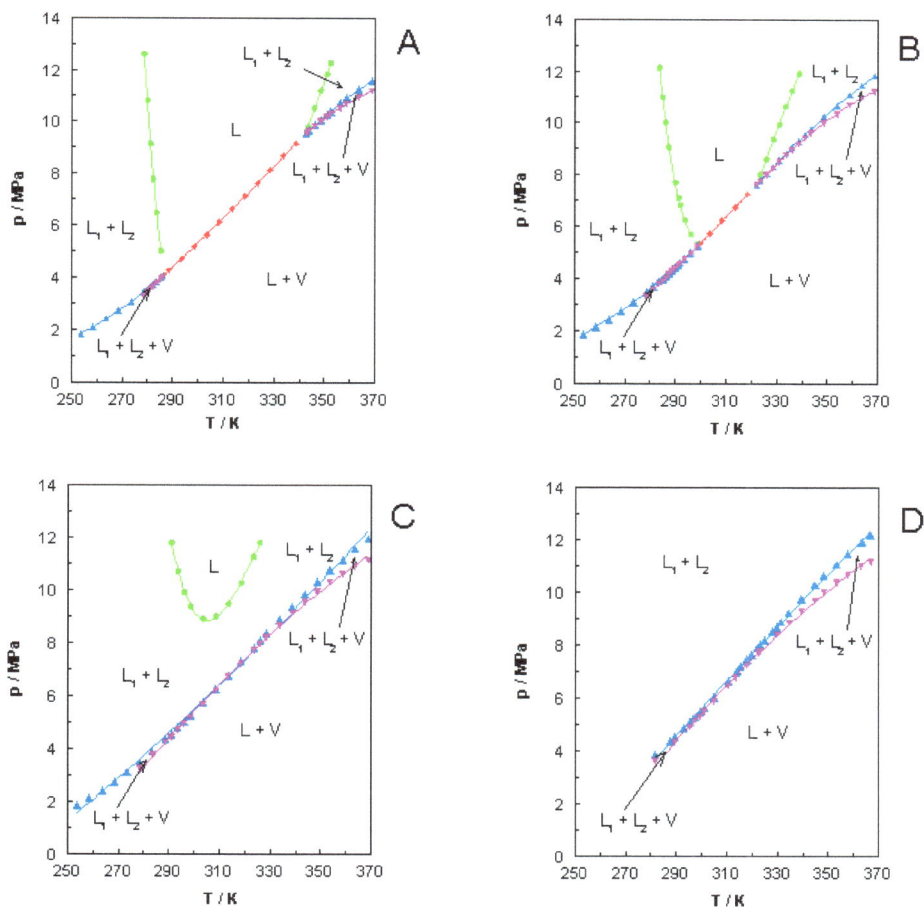

Figure 4: The miscibility switch in the ternary system CO_2 + hmim[BF$_4$] + isopropanol [46]. Concentration of hmim[BF$_4$] in isopropanol is constant at 4.74 mol% for all systems. Mol fraction of CO_2 in ternary system: A (0.5209), B (0.5410), C (0.5596) and D (0.6023).

PHASE DIAGRAMS: SYSTEMS WITH IONIC LIQUIDS

In the last years more attention has been dedicated to the investigation of the phase behavior of ionic liquid-based systems. Up to now, binary systems are by far the most studied ones, especially on the solubility of gases in ionic liquids. Different classifications of phase behavior of binary systems with ionic liquids have also arisen. Gutkowski and co-workers [48] concluded that the system 1-octyl-3-methylimidazolium tetrafluoroborate + CO_2 behaves as type III according to the classification of Scott and van Konynenburg [49]. The same conclusion applies to the systems 1-hexyl-3-methylimidazolium tetrafluoroborate + CO_2 [50]. Shiflett and Yokozeki classified mixtures of hydrofluorocarbon compounds and CO_2 as belonging to type V fluid phase behavior [51], while Shariati and coworkers identified the type III phase behavior in the system CHF_3 + bmim[PF_6] [52].

Most experimental work on the liquid-liquid equilibrium of binary systems with ionic liquids detected upper critical solution temperature (UCST) behavior [53, 54]. Recently, J. Lachwa *et al.* claimed to have found the first experimental evidence of type VII fluid phase diagram in systems with 1-alkyl-3-methylimidazolium ionic liquids and the NTf_2^- (bis{(trifluoromethyl)sulfonyl}amide anion [55]. Type VII fluid phase diagrams have been up to then, only theoretically postulated and its existence had been never confirmed experimentally.

Ternary systems ionic liquid + solute + CO_2 have been also investigated. For instance, Zhang *et al.* [56] detected the co-solvent and anti-solvent effect of CO_2 in the mixture bmim[BF_4] + water. Since water highly interferes in the properties of ionic liquids, it is always useful to know the effect of CO_2 in the mutual solubility of these compounds, as well as to understand under which conditions the homogeneous mixture can be split and water separated from the ionic liquid.

In another contribution, Aki and co-workers [57], presented the phase equilibria of different ionic liquid + organic + CO_2 mixtures, and analyzed how CO_2 influences the split of the homogeneous mixtures into two liquid phases. They concluded that both the organic and the ionic liquid have influence on the pressure and temperature conditions in which the split in phases occurs. The Lower Critical Endpoint Pressure (LCEP) and the K-point pressure of those ternary mixtures were studied based on the composition of the ionic liquid + organic solution. They found that the LCEP is dependant on both the type of organic and ionic liquid chosen, while the K-point is only dependant on the organic compound selected. Of course, this was to be expected since ionic liquids poorly dissolve in CO_2, and the K-point determines the conditions where the organic compound and the CO_2 phase become critical. In a recent analysis of this phase behavior [58], it was shown that the nomenclature LCEP and K-point is erroneous. Both points are normal phase transitions and have nothing to do with criticality.

Zhang *et al.* [59] published a study on the ternary system bmim[PF_6] + acetone + CO_2, detecting not only regions with liquid-liquid immiscibility, but also the presence of a three-phase region from 4.9 MPa up to 8.1 MPa, at a constant temperature of 313.15 K. Additionally, they confirmed that the presence of a polar compound in the mixture IL+CO_2 enhances the solubility of the ionic liquid in the supercritical phase, as was discovered previously by Wu *et al.* [38].

The first quaternary system with ionic liquids and carbon dioxide has been studied by Najdanovic-Visak *et al.* [53], where the effect of CO_2 pressure in the induction of phase changes in systems with an ionic liquid was presented. In this publication, the phase behavior of the system bmim[Tf_2N] + 1-butanol + water + CO_2 was investigated for different compositions over a temperature range from 295.6 K up to 333.15 K. According to their results, two-liquid phases are found at about 57 bars, and the increase in CO_2 concentration favors the mixing of these two liquid phases, until their complete miscibility at approximately 214 bars. The authors concluded that the pressure needed to separate the phases is also strongly dependant on the water concentration in the system. Their measurements confirm the miscibility switch phenomenon also for quaternary systems, demonstrating that this phenomenon can also be applied for systems liquid$_1$+liquid$_2$+liquid$_3$+CO_2.

IONIC LIQUIDS, CARBON DIOXIDE AND THE PHARMACEUTICAL INDUSTRY

Particularly pharmaceutical companies are facing substantial challenges to replace their troublesome processes to more environmentally friendly ones. The syntheses of drugs quite often are based on multi-step reactions involving large amounts of organic solvents and generating undesirable by-products as well. The Environmental factor (E-factor) developed by R.A. Sheldon [60, 61] measures the amount of waste (kg) generated per kilogram of product. It shows that pharmaceutical companies are the ones producing the most waste from all industry branches, from 25 to 100 kg of waste per kg of product. Part of this waste is the release of volatile organic solvents into the atmosphere.

As it is known, most active pharmaceutical ingredients are manufactured by chemical synthesis in which fine chemicals and intermediates undergo significant chemical change through a series of multi-step processes. These synthesis processes typically include the use of organic solvents and, therefore, traditionally require organic solvents for process cleaning. A growing trend exists in the industry to move away from solvent-based cleaning to aqueous cleaning whenever possible, driven by safety, regulatory and economic factors.

Since the E-factor of pharmaceutical companies is the largest found among all different industrial sectors, a reduction in the use of volatile organic solvents in drug synthesis would lead to a more efficient, less pollutant and less harmful process.

Industrial applications with new technology, however, are more likely to be applied if economic motivators exist. If economical advantages drive the adoption of neoteric solvents in industry, then environmental advantages can be expected as consequences, including reduced evaporative losses, reduced reliance on petrochemical-derived solvents, reduced hazardous waste and increased solvent recycling. The pay off for the implementation of new processes based on ionic liquids, therefore, is most likely to be attractive for industries with products that have high added values, as it is the case of medicines. The high purity of the final product required in the synthesis of drugs is another reason to justify the implementation of ionic liquids – CO_2 based processes.

REFERENCES

[1]   Earle, M.J.; Seddon, K.R. *Pure Appl. Chem.*, **2000**, 72, 1391.

[2]   Rogers, R.D.; Seddon, K.R. *Science*, **2003**, 302, 792.

[3]   Wilkes, J.S.; Levisky, J.A.; Wilson, R.A. ; Hussey, C.L. *Inorg. Chem.*, **1982,** 21(3), 1263.

[4]   Wilkes, J.S. ; Zaworotko, M.J. *J. Chem. Soc., Chem. Commun.*, **1992**, 965.

[5]   Davis Jr., J.H.; Forrester, K.J.; Merrigan, T. *Tetrahedron Letters*, **1998**, 39, 8955.

[6]   Visser, A.E.; Swatloski, R.P.; Reichert, W.M.; Mayton, R.; Sheff, S.; Wierzbicki, A.; Davis Jr, J.H.; Rogers, R.D. *Chemical Communications*, **2001**, 135.

[7]   Wasserscheid, P. *Nature*, **2006**, 439, 797.

[8]   Earle, M.J.; Esperança, J.M.S.S.; Gilea, M.A.; Canongia Lopes, J.N.; Rebelc, L.P.N.; Magee, J.W.; Seddon K.R.; Widegren, J.A. *Nature*, **2006**, 439, 831.

[9]   Imperato, G.; König, B.; Chiappe, C. *Eur. J. Org. Chem.*, **2007**, 1049.

[10]   Vu, P.D.; Boydston, A.J.; Bielawski, C.W. *Green Chem.*, **2007**, 9, 1158.

[11]   Zhou, Z.; Wang, T.; Xing, H. *Ind. Eng. Chem. Res.*, **2006**, 45, 525.

[12]   Gathergood, N.; Scammells, P.J. *Aust. J. Chem.,* **2002**, 55, 557.

[13]   Marsh, K.N.; Boxall, J.A.; Lichtenthaler, R. *Fluid Phase Equilibria*, **2004**, 219, 93

[14]   Seddon, K.R.; Stark, A.; Torres, M-J. *Pure Appl. Chem.*, **2000**, 72(12), 2275.

[15]   MacFarlane, D.R.; Forsyth, S.A.; Golding, J.; Deacon, G.B. *Green Chemistry*, **2002**, 4, 444.

[16]   Wasserscheid, P.; Keim, W. *Angew. Chem. Int. Ed.*, **2000**, 39, 3772.

[17]   Wasserscheid, P.; Welton, T. *Ionic Liquids in Synthesis*. 1st ed.; Wiley-VCH: Weinheim, *2002.*

[18]   Every, H.A.; Bishop, A.G.; MacFarlane, D.R.; Orädd, G.; Forsyth, M. *Phys. Chem Chem. Phys.*, **2004**, 6, 1758.

[19]   Jastorff, B.; Störmann, R.; Ranke, J.; Mölter, K.; Stock, F.; Oberheitmann, B.; Hoffmann, W.; Hoffmann, J.; Nüchter, M.; Ondruschka, B.; Filser, J. *Green Chemistry*, **2003**, 5, 136.

[20]   Jastorff, B.; Mölter, K.; Behrend, P.; Bottin-Weber, U.; Filser, J.; Heimers, A.; Cndruschka, B.; Ranke, J.; Schaefer, M.; Schröder, H.; Stark, A.; Stepnowski, P.; Stock, F.; Störmann, R.; Stolte, S.; Welz-Biermann, U.; Ziegert, S.; Thöming, J. *Green Chemistry*, **2005**, 7, 362.

[21]   Docherty, K.M.; Kulpa Jr., C.F. *Green Chemistry*, **2005**, 7, 185.

[22]   Stolte, S.; Arning, J.; Bottin-Weber, U.; Matzke, M.; Stock, F.; Thiele, K.; Uerdingen, M.; Welz-Biermann, U.; Jastorff, B.; Ranke, J. *Green Chem.*, **2006**, 8, 621.

[23]   Bernot, R.J.; Brueseke, M.A.; Evans-White, M.A.; Lamberti, G.A. *Environmental Toxicology and Chemistry*, **2005**, 24(1), 87.

[24]   Couling, D.J.; Bernot, R.J.; Codherty, K.M.; Dixon, J.K.; Maginn, E.J.; *Green Chemistry*, **2006**, 8, 82.

[25]   Tadros, T.F. *Applied Surfactants: Principles and Applications*; Wiley VCH, *2005.*

[26]   Colnot, T. (Merck KGaA), *Communication at the BATIL Meeting*, 6-8 May **2007**, Berlin-Germany.

[27]   Docherty, K.M.; Hebeller, S.Z.; Kulpa Jr., C.F. *Green Chemistry*, **2006**, 8, 560.

[28]   Darr, J.A.; Poliakoff, M. *Chem. Rev.*, **1999**, 99, 495.

[29]   McHugh, M.A.; Krukonis, V.J. *Supercritical Fluid Extraction: principles and practice*, 2nd ed.; Butterworth-Heinemann, 1994.

[30]   Eckert, C.A.; Knutson, B.L.; Debenedetti, P.G. *Nature*, **1996**, 383, 313.

[31]   Beckman, E.J. *The Journal of Supercritical Fluids*, **2004**, 28(2-3), 121.

[32]   Shariati, A.; Peters, C.J. *The Journal Supercritical Fluids*, **2002**, 23, 195.

[33]   Cadena, C.; Anthony, J.L.; Shah, J.K.; Morrow, T.I.; Brennecke, J.F.; Maginn, E.J.; *J. Am. Chem. Soc.*, **2004**, 126, 5300.

[34]   Blanchard, L.A.; Gu, Z.; Brennecke, J.F. *J. Phys. Chem. B*, **2001**, 105, 2437.

[35]   Aki, S.N.V.K.; Mellein, B.R.; Saurer, E.M.; Brennecke, J.F.; *J. Phys. Chem. B*, **2004**, 108, 20355.

[36]   Jessop, P.G.; Stanley, R.R.; Brown, R.A.; Eckert, C.A.; Liotta, C.L.; Ngob, T.T.; Pollet, P. *Green Chemistry*, **2003**, 5, 123.

[37]   Blanchard, L.A.; Brennecke, J.F., *Ind. Eng. Chem. Res.*, **2001**, 40(1), 287.

[38]   Wu, W.; Zhang, J.; Han, B.; Chen, J.; Liu, Z.; Jiang, T.; He, J.; Li, W. *Chem. Commun.*, **2003**, 12, 1412.

[39]   Wu, W.; Li, W.; Han, B.; Jiang, T.; Shen, D.; Zhang, Z.; Sun, D.; Wang, B. *J. Chem. Eng. Data*, **2004**, 49(6), 1597.

[40]   Peters, C.J.; Gauter, K. *Chem. Rev.*, **1999**, 99, 419.

[41]   Gauter, K.; Peters, C.J.; Scheidgen, A.L.; Schneider, G.M. *Fluid Phase Equilibria*, **2000**, 171, 127.

[42]   Scurto, A.M.; Aki, S.N.V.K.; Brennecke, J.F. *J. Am. Chem. Soc.*, **2002**, 124(35), 10276.

[43]   Scurto, A.M.; Aki, S.N.V.K.; Brennecke, J.F. *Chem. Commun.*, **2003**, 5, 572.

[44]   Lee, S.; Zhang, Y.J.; Piao, J.Y.; Yoon, H.; Song, C.E.; Choi, J.H.; Hong, J. *Chem. Commun.*, **2003**, 2624.

[45]   Kroon, M.C.; Shariati, A.; Florusse, L.J.; Peters, C.J.; van Spronsen, J.; Witkamp, G-J.; Sheldon, R.A.; Gutkowski, K.E. International Patent WO 2006/088348 A1 (2006).

[46]   Florusse, L.J.; Domingo Force, E.; Peters, C.J.; *"Fluid Phase Equilibria in the Ternary System Carbon Dioxide + Iso-propanol + 1-Hexyl-3-methylimidazolium Tetrafluoroborate"*, in preparation.

[47]   Gauter, K.; Heidemann, R.A.; Peters, C.J. *Fluid Phase Equilibria*, **1999**, 158-160, 133.

[48]   Gutkowski, K.I.; Shariati, A.; Peters, C.J. *J. Supercrit. Fluids*, **2006**, 39, 187.

[49]   van Konynenburg, P.H.; Scott, R.L. *Philos. Trans. Royal Soc. London*, **1980**, 298 A, 495.

[50]   Costantini, M.; Toussaint, V.A.; Shariati, A.; Peters, C.J.; Kikic, I. *J. Chem. Eng. Data*, **2005**, 50, 52.

[51]   Shiflett, M.B.; Yokozeki, A. *Fluid Phase Equilibria*, **2007**, 259, 210.

[52]   Shariati, A.; Gutkowski, K.; Peters, C.J. *AIChE Journal*, **2005**, 51(5), 1532.

[53]   Nadjanovic-Visak, V.; Rebelo, L.P.N.; da Ponte, M.N. *Green Chemistry*, **2005**, 7, 443.

[54]   Crosthwaite, J.M.; Aki, S.N.V.K.; Maginn, E.J.; Brennecke, J.F. *Fluid Phase Equilibria*, **2005**, 228-229, 303.

[55]   Lachwa, J.; Szydlowski, J.; Najdanovic-Visak, V.; Rebelo, L.P.N.; Seddon, K.R.; da Ponte, M.N.; Esperança, J.M.S.S.; Guedes, H.J.R. *J. Am. Chem. Soc.*, **2005**, 127, 654.

[56]   Zhang, Z.; Wu, W.; Gao, H.; Han, B.; Wang, B.; Huang, Y. *Phys. Chem. Chem. Phys.*, **2004**, 6, 5051

[57]   Aki, S.N.V.K.; Scurto, A.M.; Brennecke, J.F. *Ind. Eng. Chem. Res.*, **2006**, 45, 5574.

[58]   Kühne, E; Alfonsín, L.R; Mota Martinez, M.T.; Witkamp, G.J; Peters, C.J. *J. of Phys. Chem. B*, **2009**, 113, 6579.

[59]   Zhang, Z.; Wu, W.; Wang, B.; Chen, J.; Shen, D.; Han, B. *The Journal of Supercritical Fluids*, **2007**, 40, 1.

[60]   Sheldon, R.A. *Chem. Ind. (London)*, **1992**, 903.

[61]   Sheldon, R.A. *Pure Appl. Chem.*, **2000**, 72(7), 1233.

CHAPTER 8

Supercritical Antisolvent Fractionation of Plant Extracts

O. J. Catchpole,* N. E. Durling, J. B. Grey, W. Eltringham and S. J. Tallon

Industrial Research Limited, PO Box 31-310, Lower Hutt, New Zealand; Email: O.Catchpole@irl.cri.nz

Abstract: A recently developed continuous process entitled supercritical antisolvent fractionation is described for the fractionation of plant extract solutions using near-critical fluids to give two or more fractions containing bioactives with widely differing polarities. One fraction is insoluble in the near critical fluid and is precipitated by antisolvent behaviour, and the other fraction is soluble in the near-critical fluid and co-solvent, and is recovered by downstream pressure reduction. With two-stage pressure reduction, two fractions may be obtained. The extract solutions are obtained by the prior extraction of plant material using ethanol/water mixtures. The process has been tested on a wide variety of plant extract solutions, including those obtained from sage, olive leaf, hop marc, grape marc, black currant, propolis, Echinacea, St Johns Wort, and onion biomass. The key parameters controlling the process are the solvent composition, concentration of dissolved solids in the solution, flow rate ratio of solution to near-critical fluid, temperature and pressure. In general, the separation between highly polar bioactives, which are recovered in the insoluble fraction (raffinate); and low to medium polarity fractions, which are recovered in the extract fraction(s) is maximised at low soluble solids, water contents in the feed solution ≤ 30 % by mass, and flow rate ratios of feed to CO_2 of ≤ 30 % when using CO_2. The process is simple to scale up, and has been performed from a laboratory to demonstration scale for propolis tincture.

INTRODUCTION

The extraction of high value products from plant and animal raw materials with supercritical fluids has technical limitations. The most widely used supercritical fluid, CO_2, can only extract low to medium polarity, low molecular weight compounds. In addition, the raw material usually needs to be dried before extraction. The range of compounds that are extractable are improved if co-solvents are used, but the improvement is small. In contrast, ethanol and ethanol/water mixtures are solvents that enable a broad range of compounds to be extracted. These solvents have been used for centuries to extract a wide range of plant materials. Here, we describe a versatile process for the fractionation of such solvent solutions resulting from an upstream extraction or processing operation. This new process has been entitled "Supercritical Antisolvent Fractionation Technology" or SAFT. The process utilises the poor solubility of water and polar compounds in supercritical fluids to produce an insoluble fraction; and the solvent power of the supercritical fluid and partially dissolved co-solvent to produce at least one extract fraction. A schematic of the process is shown in Fig. **1**. The process is not limited to CO_2 being the near-critical fluid; dimethyl ether enables largely aqueous streams to also be processed. The SAFT process has so far been applied to the production of polyunsaturated fatty acids from fish and plant oils [1,2]; the production of flavonoid concentrates from propolis [3]; the extraction of lipids from aqueous lipid/protein streams including dairy and egg yolk [4-6]; and the fractionation of plant and animal extract solutions as shown in Table **1** below [7] and from recent work. The table includes examples of the extraction of dry materials (sage, olive leaf, grape marc); wet materials (onions); and materials that have been previously extracted with supercritical CO_2 (hop marc, grape seed). The plant raw materials contain a mixture of desirable compounds covering a range of polarities. Table **1** shows the desirable, or target compounds for the plant materials investigated.

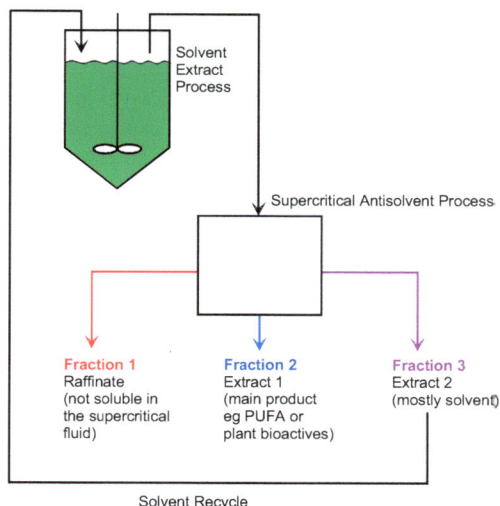

Figure 1: Supercritical antisolvent fractionation process schematic.

Ana Rita C. Duarte & Catarina M. M. Duarte (Eds)

Table 1: Target compounds for extraction *pre-extracted using supercritical CO_2.

Plant material	Low polarity	Medium polarity	High polarity
Sage	oleoresin	carnosol, carnosic acid	rosemarinic acid
Echinacea	alkamides		chichoric acid
St Johns Wort	hyperforin		hypericin
Olive leaf	vitamin E	oleuropein	flavonoids
Grape seed	grape oil*		anthocyanins
Grape skin	waxes		anthocyanins
Hops	hop acids*	xanthohumol, resins	flavonoids
Propolis	cinnamic acids	aglycone flavonoids	polyphenolic oligomers
Onions	sulphur compounds		flavonoids

In this work, we describe the use of the SAFT process in detail for the solvent extraction and subsequent supercritical antisolvent fractionation of sage and onion. The extraction and pre-processing of the feed materials is described, followed by SAFT processing.

EXPERIMENTAL

Materials

Functional Dried sage leaf and stem was supplied by Crop and Food Research Ltd (NZ). Olive leaf was supplied by Mende Biotech Ltd (NZ), and air dried on-site at IRL. Onions and onion waste was supplied by Crop and Food Research Ltd (NZ). Echinacea leaf and tops tinctures were supplied by Extracts NZ Ltd. Hop marc previously extracted using supercritical CO_2 (type Pacific Gem) was supplied by Extracts Solutions Ltd and The Horticultural Research Institute (NZ). Grape marc (seeds and skins, Pinot Noir) were supplied freeze dried by Auckland University, and were separated into seeds and skins by Crop and Food Research (NZ). Black currant marc and tincture was supplied by Nutrizeal/Tasman Extracts Ltd (NZ). CO_2 was purchased from BOC (NZ) Ltd. Dimethyl ether (DME) was purchased from Aerosol Products Ltd. Anhydrous ethanol was purchased from Barwell Pacific. Water was distilled on-site. HP-20 resin was purchased from Sigma-Aldrich.

Solvent Extraction and Pre-Processing

Solvent extraction of plant materials was performed at a laboratory scale using glass beakers; and at a pilot scale using 20 litre pre-weighed plastic buckets. The method is described for pilot scale extractions. Laboratory scale extraction methodology is described elsewhere [8,9]. Dry plant material was ground in a Wiley knife mill. A known mass of plant material was then added to the extraction vessel, followed by a known mass of hydro-alcoholic solvent. A stainless steel heating coil was then inserted into the bucket, followed by the overhead stirrer paddle. Water at the desired extraction temperature was passed through the inside of the heating coil. A temperature probe was suspended in the extraction solvent mixture to monitor the temperature. The solvent and plant mixture was stirred at a sufficient rate to suspend the solids. After stirring for a measured extraction time, the stirrer was stopped and removed along with the heating coil. The contents of the bucket were then vacuum filtered on a Büchner funnel to separate the solvent solution from the solids. The residual solids and recovered solvent solution were weighed to determine the solvent loss and perform mass balances. A small sample of the solvent solution was evaporated to dryness to obtain the solids content. When wet or fresh plant material was extracted, it was first ground in an Urschel knife mill and/or an industrial mincer. The ground plant material was then passed through a Vetter dewatering screw press (dejuicer) to reduce the water content of the solids and thus reduce the ethanol required to achieve a desired high ethanol to water solvent ratio. The solids and juice were collected in separate, pre-weighed buckets. A small sample of the feed and dejuiced solids was air dried overnight in a forced convection oven at 40 - 60°C to determine their moisture contents. Solvent extraction was then performed as described above for dry materials.

Supercritical Antisolvent Fractionation

The supercritical antisolvent process was carried out at both a laboratory scale, and at a pilot scale in the apparatus shown schematically in Fig. **2**, and then passed through either a static mixer or nozzle housed inside the vessel. The part of the solution that is not soluble in CO_2, herein referred to as the raffinate, was sprayed onto the bottom of the extraction vessel, and recovered through valve EXV1. This stream was largely aqueous, with dissolved high polarity/high molecular mass compounds. Meanwhile, the extract phase, consisting of CO_2 and a large portion of the ethanol from the feed solution, left the top of the extraction vessel and then passed through pressure reduction valve CV1 and another heat exchanger (not shown). Alternatively, the extract phase left EX1 and was then mixed with an aqueous phase supplied by pump LP2 before entering the second antisolvent fractionation vessel EX2 to perform a water wash of the extract phase. Again, a second raffinate phase was recovered from the bottom of the vessel through valve EXV2, while the new extract phase was recovered from the top of the vessel, and then passed through pressure reduction valve CV1. The pressure was then usually reduced to an intermediate pressure P2, usually set to a pressure slightly above the critical pressure for CO_2-ethanol at the first separator temperature. A portion of the extract was precipitated into the bottom of the first separation vessel SV1 and recovered through valve EV4 and optionally flash vessel SV4. This extract tended to be solutes that have a poor solubility in pure CO_2, but reasonable solubility in mixtures of CO_2 + ethanol. Finally, the extract phase and remaining dissolved solutes left the top of the first separation vessel SV1 and then passed through a second pressure reduction valve CV2 and heat exchanger HX3 to reduce the pressure to the recirculation/cylinder pressure P3. The remaining extract including the bulk of the ethanol co-solvent was precipitated into the second separator SV2, and recovered through valve EV5 and optionally flash vessel SV5. The same set-up was also used for antisolvent experiments using dimethyl ether for feed streams that had high water contents and/or high amounts of medium polarity materials.

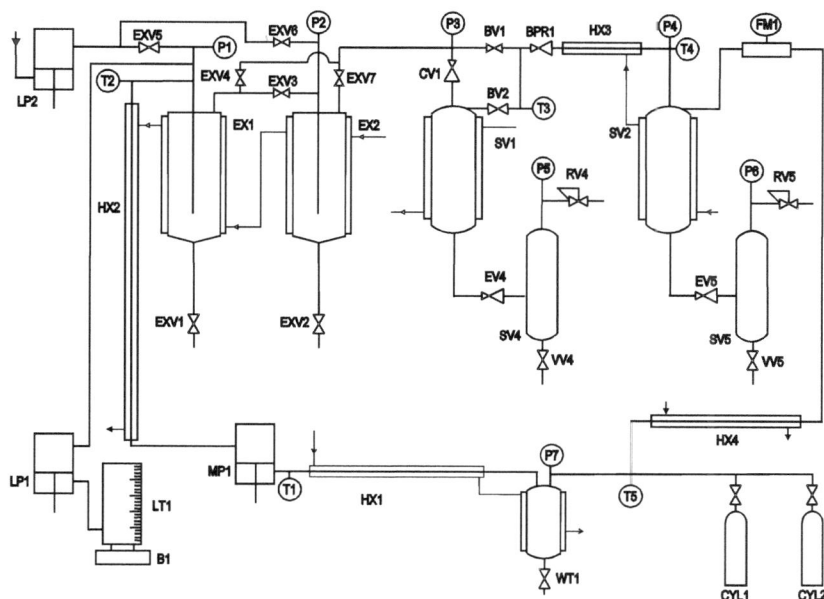

Figure 2: Schematic of pilot scale supercritical antisolvent fractionation plant

CO_2 Extraction of Plant Materials

Hop marc pellet and powder were supplied already extracted using supercritical CO_2 by Nutrizeal Ltd (NZ). Pilot scale extraction of grape seed and grape skin was performed on the same pilot scale apparatus shown in Fig. **1**, using a pressure of 300 bar and temperature of 313 K. The oil yield obtained from ground seeds was ~ 10 % by mass, which is within the range reported by other workers [10,11]. The extract yield obtained from skins was very low, at around 1 % by mass. This extract was very waxy, and solid at room temperature. The extraction of sage [12,13], Echinacea and St Johns Wort [14] using CO_2 has been reported previously, giving yields of around 2-3 % of mainly essential oil and flavour compounds; 2-3 % of an extract enriched in alkamides; and 6-7 % of an extract enriched in hyperforin respectively. Dry olive leaf was extracted at a laboratory scale, giving a yield of around 1-2 % of waxy material containing some tocopherol. A general procedure for partially dewatering fresh feed materials and then extracting the dewatered residue has been described, including onions [15], where the yield of extract on a fresh onion basis was ~ 0.1 % by mass.

RESULTS AND DISCUSSION

The combined process of hydro-ethanolic extraction of plant material, followed by supercritical antisolvent fractionation was applied to a number of plant materials. The separation of rosmarinic acid from carnosol/carnosic acid, and oleoresin was successfully achieved for sage. The separation of oleuropein (and flavonoids) from vitamin E, leaf waxes and chlorophyll was successfully demonstrated for olive leaf. Oleuropein was then further concentrated from the raffinate using DME. The concentration of xanthohumol was successfully achieved from hop marc, as was the concentration of polyphenolics from onions. The separation efficiency of the SAFT process depends on the prior solvent extraction of the plant material; phase equilibrium in the antisolvent fractionation and separators; and the process parameters flow rate ratio of solution to CO_2, and the concentration of feed solids in the solution. The influence of these parameters on the separation efficiency is discussed below, using mainly sage and propolis antisolvent fractionation as model examples. The concentration of water in the feed solution, the temperature and pressure also have an effect on the process but are not discussed here.

Solvent Extraction of Plant Materials

The solvent extraction and pre-processing of the raw material is critical to the downstream SAFT process. The aim of the solvent extraction process is to optimize the extraction of the desired components, within a solvent composition range that is amenable to SAFT processing. When using CO_2 as the antisolvent, the usable composition range has at least 60 % by mass ethanol. At an industrial scale, it is important to minimise the amount of solvent used whilst still achieving the desired extract spectrum, minimise the losses of solvent in the plant material within practical limits of available equipment, and to recycle the solvent where possible from the antisolvent fractionation process. Here, results achieved for the hydro-alcoholic solvent extraction of dry sage up to a pilot scale are discussed. Sage is a model plant material as it contains a mixture of desirable compounds ranging from essential oil/flavour compounds with low polarity, to fat soluble antioxidants of medium polarity (carnosol and carnosic acid) to water soluble antioxidants of high polarity (rosemarinic acid). The optimum conditions for the hydro-ethanolic extraction of sage were investigated in some detail [8]. The parameters investigated included particle size, extraction time, extraction temperature, solvent to feed ratio, and solvent composition. The optimal solvent composition for extraction of all three components in a stirred tank apparatus is shown in Fig. **3**.

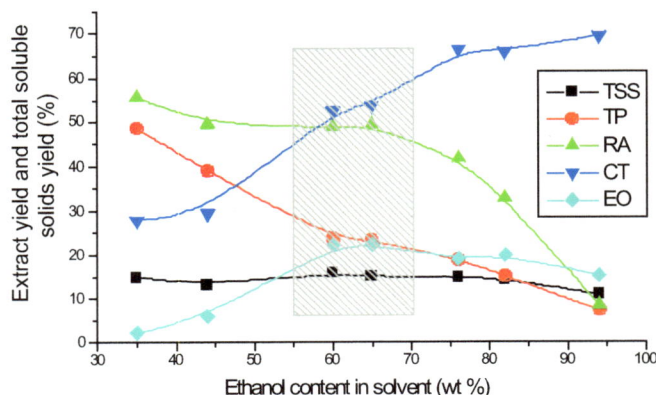

Figure 3: Optimal hydro-alcoholic solvent composition for extraction of sage (see text below for legend details)

The grey hatched area in Fig. **3** shows the optimal solvent composition to achieve good yields of essential oil and flavour components (EO); lipophilic antioxidants belonging to the carnosic acid family (CT); rosmarinic acid (RA); total phenolics (TP) and total soluble solids (TSS). We have found that the optimal solvent composition is also in the range 60 – 80 % ethanol for the extraction of other dry feed materials including hop marc, grape seed and skin, olive leaf, St Johns Wort, Echinacea and propolis. Typically, the ratio of solvent to solids was in the range 4-6:1

The hydro-alcoholic process can also be performed on materials that initially have high moisture contents. Here, we use onions as an example, which have feed moisture contents of the order 90 % by mass. The onions are first passed through a mincer, and then through a dejuicing screw press, to reduce the water content. Previous work has shown that there is little loss of the desired compounds into the juice fraction [15]. In some cases the solids were then subjected to centrifuging, to remove further juice. When the screw press alone was used, between 45 – 60 % of the mass of the onions is removed as the juice. When centrifuging was also used, up to 73 % of the mass was removed as a juice fraction. The solids were then extracted with ethanol, to give an extract solution containing approximately 70 % ethanol, and the balance co-extracted water. The extract solution also contained sulphur compounds, oligosaccharides, and flavonoids.

Phase equilibrium for CO_2-ethanol-water system

Understanding the phase equilibria of the antisolvent fractionation process is essential for implementation of the technology at a large scale. The phase equilibria at the antisolvent conditions, first separator conditions, and second separator conditions all need to be considered. Ideally, the process should be operated with a high ratio of feed solution to CO_2 to maximise throughput, the first separator at conditions where very little ethanol is precipitated, and the second separator where the bulk of the ethanol is separated. However, these conditions are not mutually compatible, when the process is operated over the normal temperature range for supercritical CO_2 extraction processes, of 313 to 363 K. The phase equilibria for the ethanol/water/CO_2 system has been measured and modelled over a range of temperatures and pressures by us [10] and others [11-16] over the conditions relevant to supercritical antisolvent fractionation. While the phase equilibria is influenced by the presence of dissolved solutes, the behaviour of the three component mixture with respect to pressure, temperature and feed composition usefully illustrates the more complex situation. At the extremes of three component mixtures, water and CO_2 are almost immiscible; ethanol and CO_2 are completely miscible at moderate pressures for a given temperature over the temperature range 313 – 353 K [23], and water and ethanol are completely miscible.

Fig. **4** shows the three component phase equilibrium on a mass basis at 313 K, and tie lines for typical extraction/antisolvent and separator conditions for 10 % and 20 % mass ratio of feed solution to CO_2 with a 70:30 ethanol/water mixture at 200 bar; first and second separator at 90 bar and 50 bar respectively) and a close-up of the CO_2-rich phase for these conditions. The two-phase region increases in size as the pressure reduces at constant temperature, and at the second separator conditions, the two-phase region expands to also include the ethanol/CO_2 binary mixture. This is to be expected, as the CO_2 is now a moderately dense gas. Decreasing the ratio of feed to CO_2 results in increasing levels of water in both the raffinate and first separator liquid phases. The liquid phase in the final separator is ethanol close to its azeotropic composition. As the feed to CO_2 ratio increases and the amount of ethanol in the raffinate increases, the partitioning of solutes that are slightly soluble in CO_2 + ethanol begins to favour the raffinate phase. Also of interest is that the liquid phase for both the first and second separator has a high concentration of CO_2 dissolved in it, at between 30 and 40 % by mass. The first separator is normally operated at conditions just above the critical point forethanol/CO_2 binary mixtures, typically around 90 bar at 313 K; and 110 bar at 333 K. The second separator is operated at dense gas conditions. Here, there is still a small amount of ethanol that is co-extracted and recirculated in the gas phase. When the process is performed at a commercial scale, the CO_2 should be partially recovered by operating secondary separators (as shown for the pilot plant schematic) in which the pressure is further reduced and/or the temperature increased to lower the solubility of the CO_2 in the liquid phase, or there will be large losses of CO_2 from the process.

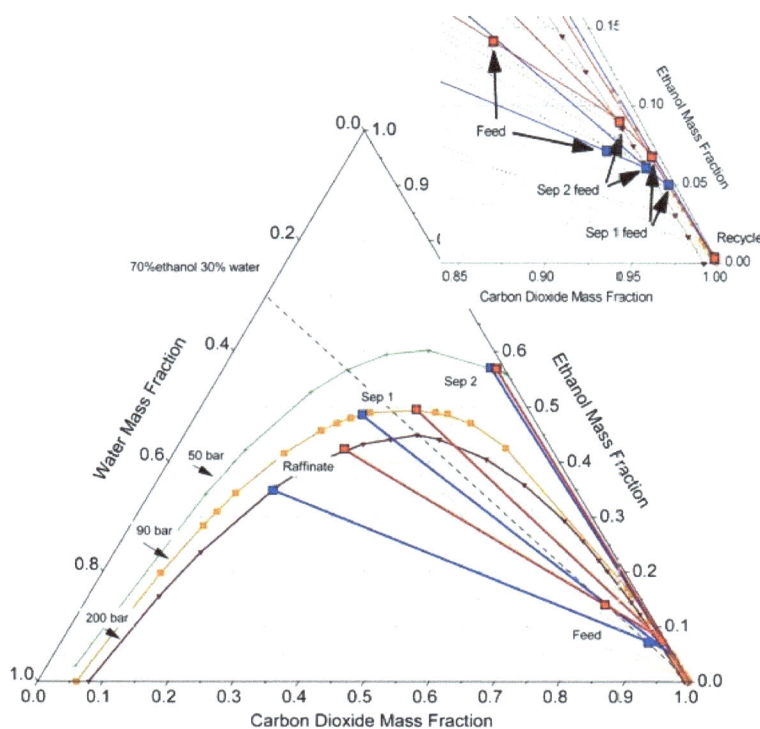

Figure 4: Phase equilibrium for CO_2-ethanol-water systems at 200 bar (brown line), 90 bar (orange line) and 50 bar (green line) at 313 K and tie lines for feed mass ratios of 10 (blue lines) and 20 % (red lines)

Ratio of Feed Solution to CO_2

It is desirable to use as high a ratio of feed solution to CO_2 as possible, as this maximises the throughput for a given size of CO_2 plant. However, the ratio cannot be increased indefinitely, as the separation performance diminishes for medium polarity components that are soluble in CO_2 + co-solvent mixtures. Additionally, losses of CO_2 in the product streams become very high, as explained in the phase equilibrium section; and losses of ethanol into the raffinate stream increase. In contrast to medium polarity constituents, low polarity (CO_2-soluble) constituents are recovered in the extract; and high polarity (CO_2 + ethanol insoluble) constituents are recovered in the raffinate at all flow rate ratios. The solvent that is co-extracted by CO_2 is largely ethanol, with the amount of water also co-extracted increasing with increasing pressure at fixed temperature, in a manner analogous to water/ethanol mixtures [16]. As the ratio of co-solvent to CO_2 increases beyond a certain level, the near-critical fluid phase after dissolution of ethanol becomes a sub-critical liquid. The recovery of medium polarity constituents is then determined almost completely by their solubility in CO_2 + co-solvent mixture, and the extent to which they partition between the raffinate and near-critical fluid phase. The solubility when in the sub-critical region is almost completely dependent upon the concentration of the co-solvent in CO_2, and is hardly affected by pressure (as long as the pressure exceeds the mixture critical point), as shown in previous work for the solubility of urea in CO_2 + ethanol mixtures [24], and the solubility of propolis flavonoids in CO_2 + ethanol [3]. The recovery and fraction concentrations are described for the supercritical antisolvent fractionation of sage extract solutions for three component groups: rosmarinic acid (RA), carnosic acid-type compounds (CA), and essential oil (EO). Fig. **5** show the recovery of these three component groups in the raffinate (R), first (S1) and second (S2) separator based on the amounts in the feed solvent solution; and the concentration of the three component groups in the same fractions for 3 feed to CO_2 ratios:

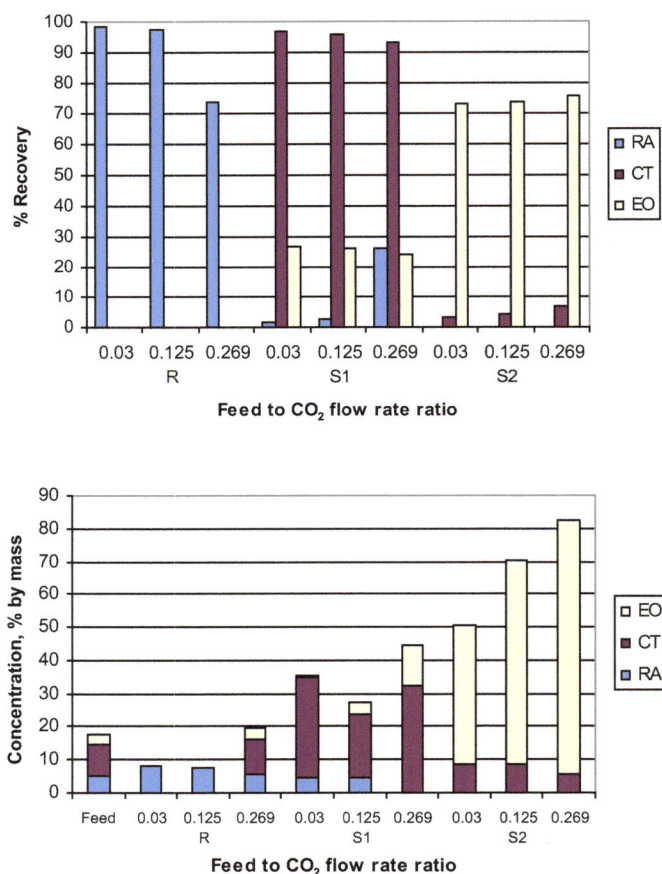

Figure 5: Recovery (top graph) and concentration (bottom graph) of key sage extract components in raffinate (R), first separator (S1) and second separator (S2) products

There is very good separation between all three groups of components. As the flow rate ratio increases, we find that there is increasing carry over of rosmarinic acid into the first separator due to an increase in its solubility in CO_2 + ethanol, and an increase in the amount of carnosic acid-type compounds that are carried over to the second separator, also due to their increasing solubility in CO_2 + ethanol at the first separator operating conditions. The solubility of carnosic acid in supercritical CO_2 + ethanol co-solvent has been measured [25]. The solubility increases exponentially with a linear increase in ethanol co-solvent concentration at a fixed pressure and temperature, and so the carry over into the second separator would be expected at high flow rate ratios and thus high concentrations of ethanol in CO_2. As the ratio of feed solution to CO_2 is increased, the mass transfer limitations of the static mixer used at the pilot scale may also result in reduced separation performance. A countercurrent spray or packed column approach can be used instead, but may instead result in phase separation issues including foaming inside the antisolvent fractionation vessel.

Dissolved Solids Concentration in Feed Solution

As the concentration of dissolved solids in the feed increases, the phase equilibria of the ethanol-water-dissolved solids mixture with CO_2 deviates increasingly from the model system ethanol-water-CO_2. When the feed solution contains high levels of polar compounds relative to medium and low polarity compounds, increasing the overall dissolved solids concentration results in a decrease in separation performance. At the very high solids content extreme, the separation achievable reduces to that obtained by using CO_2 or CO_2 with a small concentration of co-solvent from dry extract. As with the ratio of feed solution to CO_2, the recovery of medium polarity compounds is most affected by a change in solids concentration. Figs. **6**, **7** and **8** shows the recovery of key components in raffinate and separator fractions from laboratory and pilot scale trials performed on propolis tinctures; and laboratory scale trials performed on sage and olive leaf extract solutions.

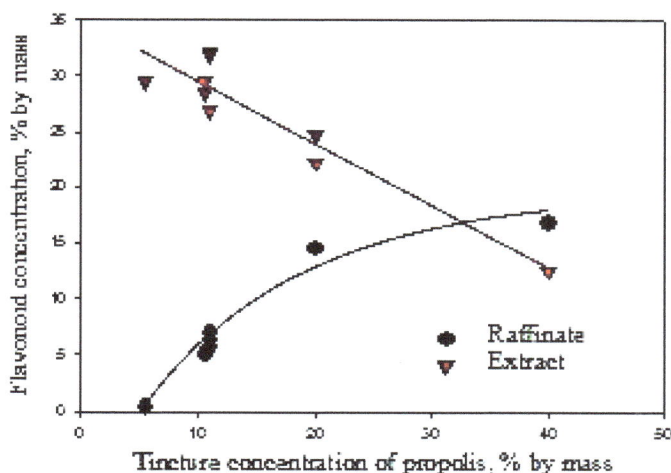

Figure 6: Propolis flavonoids concentration in the main extract and raffinate fraction as a function of the tincture concentration of dissolved propolis solids.

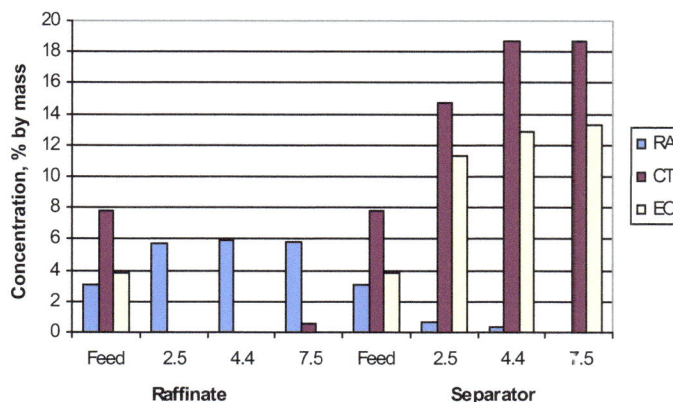

Figure 7: Concentration of rosmarinic acid (RA), carnosic acid type compounds (CT) and essential oil (EO) as a function of feed solids concentration in the raffinate and extract (separator) products

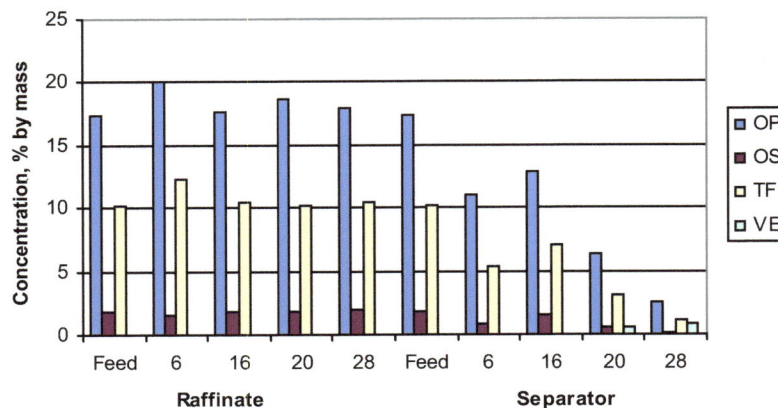

Figure 8: Concentration of oleuropein (OP), oleuroside (OS), total flavonoids (TF), and vitamin E (VE) as a function of feed solids concentration in the raffinate and extract (separator) products

In general, the recovery of polar bioactives into the raffinate, and non-polar bioactives into the separator is not affected by the solids concentration over the range investigated. With olive leaf, the bulk of the bioactive compounds are polar and not extractable using CO_2 + ethanol. The recovery of the medium polarity compounds into the separator (aglycone flavonoids in the case of propolis, and carnosic acid–type compounds for sage) decreases with increasing solids concentration.

However, the concentration of these compounds in the extract increases over the small feed solids concentration investigated. Rosmarinic acid concentrations decrease in the extract with increasing feed solids concentration. With olive leaf, oleuropein and olive leaf flavonoids have some limited solubility in CO_2 + ethanol. The recovery of these compounds into the extract phase decreases sharply with increasing solids concentration above 16 % dissolved solids.

CONCLUSIONS

A new separation process has been devised which incorporates the low cost, low technology benefits of ethanol/water extraction with fractionation of the extract solutions using near critical fluids to produce at least two fractions with added value. In comparison, the ethanol/water extraction process gives only one broad spectrum product; and supercritical extraction gives only a non-polar extract. The overall process, entitled supercritical antisolvent fractionation technology, has been demonstrated on a large number of plant materials, including sage, olive leaf, hop marc, grape marc, black currant, propolis, Echinacea, and St Johns Wort. The separation performance depends on the solvent composition of the upstream hydro-alcoholic solvent extraction process, the ratio of feed solution to supercritical fluid, the feed solids concentration, and the pressures and temperatures used for the antisolvent and separator stages. The technology is relatively simple to scale-up, and processing has been performed at laboratory, pilot and demonstration scale for some materials. The supercritical antisolvent fractionation process is completely continuous, and the cost of the supercritical extraction plant with a given CO_2 recirculation rate is low relative to an equivalent plant for extracting solid materials. Similarly, the upstream solvent extraction process is very simple, and can consist of stirred tanks, pumps and filters that operate at close to atmospheric pressure.

REFERENCES

[1]   Catchpole OJ, MacKenzie AN, Grey, JB. Improvements in or Relating to Separation Technology, NZ Patent 518504; WO03089399, priority date **2002**
[2]   Catchpole OJ, Tallon SJ, Eltringham WE, Grey JB, Fenton KA, Vagi EM, Vyssotski MV, MacKenzie AN, Ryan J, Zhu Z., *J Supercrit Fluids*, **2008**; 47, 591-597
[3]   Catchpole OJ, Grey JB, Mitchell KA, Lan JS, Supercritical antisolvent fractionation of propolis tincture. *J Supercrit Fluids*, **2004**; 29, 97-106
[4]   Fletcher KA, Fletcher A, Catchpole OJ, Grey JB, Improvements to Separation Technology NZ Patent 523920, WO2004066744 priority date **2003**

[5]   Tallon SJ, Catchpole OJ, Grey JB, Fenton K, Fletcher K, Fletcher AJ, *Chem Eng Technol*, **2007**; 30(4), 501-510

[6]   Catchpole OJ, Tallon SJ, Grey JB, Fletcher K, Fletcher AJ. *J. Supercrit Fluids*, **2008**; 45(3), 314-321

[7]   Catchpole OJ, Durling NE, Grey JB, Improvements in or relating to separation technology NZ Patent Application 545146, WO2007091901, priority date **2006**

[8]   Durling NE, Catchpole OJ, Grey JB, Webby RF, Mitchell KA, Foo LY, Perry NB, Burgess EJ., *Food Chemistry*, **2007**; 101, 1434-1441

[9]   Durling NE, Catchpole OJ, Grey JB, Mendiola JA, Webby RF, Fenton KA, Mitchell KA., *Food Chemistry*, **2009** (in press)

[10]   Gomez AM, Lopez CP, Ossa EM., *Chem Eng J*, **1996**; 61, 227

[11]   Beveridge THJ, Girard B, Kopp T, Drover JCG., *J Ag Food Chem*, **2005**; 53, 1799

[12]   Catchpole OJ, Grey JB, Smallfield BM, *ACS Symposium Series 670*, **1997**, p 76

[13]   Catchpole OJ, Grey JB, Smallfield BM, *J Supercrit Fluids*, **1996**, 9(4), 273

[14]   Catchpole OJ, Perry NB, da Silva BMT, Grey JB, Smallfield BM., *J. Supercritical Fluids*, **2002**; 22, 129-138

[15]   Catchpole OJ, Smallfield BM, Dyer PJ, Grey JB, McNamara C, Perry NB, Durling NE, 7th Italian Conference/9th European Meeting on Supercritical Fluids and Their Applications, Trieste, Italy, CD Rom, **2004**, 14-16 June.

[16]   Durling NE, Catchpole OJ, Tallon SJ, Grey JB., *Fluid Phase Equilibria*, **2007**; 252, 103-113

[17]   Gilbert ML, Paulaitis ME, *J. Chem. Eng. Data*, **1986**; 31, 296-298.

[18]   Hirohama S, Takatsuka T, Miyamoto S, Muto T, *J Chem Eng Japan*, **1993**, 26, 408-415.

[19]   Takishima S,Saiki K, Arai K, Saito S, *J Chem Eng Japan* **1986**, 19, 48-56

[20]   de la Ossa EM, Brandani V, Del Re G, Di Giacomo G, Ferri E, *Fluid Phase Equilib*, **1990**, 56, 325-340.

[21]   Yao S, Guan Y, Zhu Z, *Fluid Phase Equilib.*, **1994**, 99, 249-259.

[22]   Lim JS, Lee YY, Chun HS, *J Supercrit Fluids*, **1994**, 7, 219-230.

[23]   Yeo SD, Park SJ, Kim JW, Kim JC, *J Chem Eng Data*, **2000**; 45, 932-935

[24]   Catchpole OJ, Tallon SJ, Dyer PJ, Lan JS, Jensen B, Rasmussen OK, Grey JB., *Fluid Phase Equilibria*, **2005**, 237, 212-218

[25]   Cháfer A, Fornari T, Berna A, Ibañez E, Reglero G., *J Supercrit Fluids*, **2005**, 34, 323-329

CHAPTER 9

Mathematical Modelling of Supercritical Fluid Extraction

H. Sovová*

Institute of Chemical Process Fundamentals of the ASCR, Rozvojová 135, 16502 Prague, Czech Republic; Email: SOVOVA@icpf.cas.cz

Abstract: The kinetics of supercritical fluid extraction of valuable substances from plants depends on both extract solubility in the solvent (or phase equilibrium between the matrix and the solvent) and mass transfer resistances, particularly the resistance inside vegetable material. Different mathematical models for supercritical fluid extraction have been published in the last decades and it can be therefore difficult to choose the most suitable model for particular extraction. In this chapter, simple criteria based on time constants of mass transfer and characteristic time of equilibrium extraction are presented, two most frequent types of models for supercritical extraction from plants are mentioned with references to the literature, and the factors influencing scale-up of the process are discussed.

INTRODUCTION

Medicinal and aromatic plants and other natural products are important sources of valuable substances. These substances are often labile and therefore mild methods should be applied to isolate them from the plants. Supercritical fluid extraction (SFE) is particularly suited for such isolation as it does not expose the substances to high temperatures and is relatively fast due to outstanding transport properties of supercritical fluids. The most frequent supercritical solvent is carbon dioxide, which is as a "green" solvent much more acceptable than toxic conventional organic solvents.

The pressurised solvent circulates in extraction equipment between an extractor containing a fixed bed of plant particles, where the extract dissolves at supercritical conditions, and a separator, where the solvent is expanded to gaseous state and the extract precipitates at reduced solvent power and is collected. Thus, it is a continuous process with respect to the solvent and a batch process with respect to the plant material. Use of two or three extractors enables a continuous operation while the exhausted plant material in one of the extractors is substituted by fresh one, and two or three separators operated in series at individually adjusted pressures and temperatures enable a partial fractionation of extract on the basis of different solubility of its components.

A correct adjustment of pressures and temperatures in the extractor and in separators, solvent flow rate and extraction time is crucial for the efficiency of the process. It is therefore important to understand the processes in both parts of the equipment.

Especially the mechanisms of extraction, on which this chapter is focused, are variable in accordance with variable properties of plant materials.

As carbon dioxide is by far the most frequently applied supercritical solvent in the extraction from plants, all examples of extraction and values of model parameters in this chapter concern the extraction with carbon dioxide, while mathematical relations are of general validity.

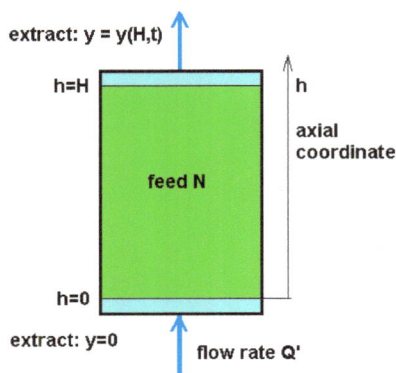

Figure 1: Scheme of cylindrical extractor with a fixed bed of particles and a continuous solvent flow.

The easily measurable variables of mathematical models for the extraction are indicated in Fig. **1**. It is the amount of material fed into the extractor, the solvent flow rate, which is maintained constant during the whole extraction run, and the concentration of extract in the solution flowing out of the extractor; its concentration in the solvent flowing into the extractor is assumed to be zero.

To describe local mass transfer rates inside the cylindrical extraction vessel, axial coordinate identical with the main direction of solvent flow is used in the models.

The extraction kinetics is characterised by extraction curves, showing the dependence of extraction yield on either extraction time, t, or solvent-to-feed ratio (the mass of solvent passed through the extractor divided by the mass of feed), q. The slope of extraction curve $e = e(q)$ is equal to instantaneous extract concentration $y(H,t)$, expressed in terms of mass of extract *per* mass of solvent. The slope of extraction curve $e = e(t)$ is equal to the product of outlet concentration and specific mass flow rate:

$$\frac{de}{dt} = q'y(H,t) \qquad (1)$$

Thus, modelling the extraction kinetics means modelling the outlet concentration $y(H,t)$ developed as a result of mass transfer from the solid phase to the fluid phase inside the extractor. The most comprehensive review on different mathematical models for SFE from plants is probably the recent paper on modelling the extraction from oilseeds [1]; another extensive survey of mathematical models is a part of a review paper published on SFE of essential oils by Reverchon [2]. Different types of SFE models were systematically classified by Al-Jabari [3]. Mathematical models for SFE presented in the literature are nowadays counted in tens and thus criteria are needed to choose a proper model for given extraction. Such criteria, frequent models, and scale-up from laboratory extraction equipment are discussed in this chapter.

MASS BALANCE EQUATIONS

The extractor is for mathematical treatment divided into finite difference volume elements of height Δh. Mass balances of the extract are written and re-arranged so that differential mass balance equations result when making $\Delta h \to 0$ and $\Delta t \to 0$. The mass balance for the fluid phase flowing through the extraction bed with interstitial velocity u is then:

$$\varepsilon\rho_f\left(\frac{\partial y}{\partial t} + u\frac{\partial y}{\partial h}\right) = j \,, y(h,t=0) = y_0, y(h=0,t) = 0 \qquad (2)$$

where $t = 0$ at the moment when the solvent just begins flowing out of the extractor. The mass balance for the solid phase is:

$$(1-\varepsilon)\rho_s\frac{\partial x}{\partial t} = -j \,, x(h,t=0) = x_0 \qquad (3)$$

The amount of extract that flows from plant particles to the solvent phase in unit volume of extraction bed and in unit time is directly proportional to the fluid phase mass transfer coefficient, specific surface area, and the difference between the extract concentrations at particle surface and in bulk fluid (driving force):

$$j = k_f a_0 \rho_f\left(y^+ - y\right) \qquad (4)$$

The scheme valid for fluid phase can be analogously applied to the solid phase:

$$j = k_s a_0 \rho_s\left(x - x^+\right) \qquad (5)$$

A more precise description of extract diffusion through the particle to its surface is based on Fick's law, characterised by effective diffusivity, D_{ef}, requires a definition of particle shape, and uses a spatially variable concentration inside the particle, c_s. For a sphere of radius R the respective equations are:

$$ j = -a_0 D_{ef} \left. \frac{\partial c_s}{\partial r} \right|_{r=R}, \quad a_0 = \frac{3(1-\varepsilon)}{R}, \quad \frac{\partial c_s}{\partial t} = \frac{D_{ef}}{r^2} \frac{\partial}{\partial r}\left(r^2 \frac{\partial c_s}{\partial r} \right). \quad (5a) $$

The initial distribution of extract between the fluid and solid phases fulfils mass balance constraint:

$$ \varepsilon \rho_f y_0 = (1-\varepsilon)\rho_s (x_u - x_0) \quad (6) $$

When the solvent flow begins immediately after pressurization of the extractor, $y_0 = 0$ can be assumed. When a period of static extraction with extraction pressure and temperature maintained in the extractor without solvent flow precedes the solvent flow out of the extractor, phase equilibrium $y_0 = y^*(x_0)$ is usually assumed to be established at $t = 0$. Generally, any value of y_0 between 0 and $y^*(x_0)$ can be applied in the models. The kinetics of static extraction can be modelled separately, as Al-Jabari [3] suggests.

Equations (1)-(6) together with a relationship between concentrations x^+, y^+ at particle surface and with equilibrium relationship constitute mathematical model for SFE. Generally, the equations have to be solved numerically to give extraction curves, which are compared with experimental curves $e(t)$ or $e(q)$. After adjustment of model parameters to fit the data measured on small-scale equipment, the model should be able to predict extractor performance for any size of extraction equipment. However, as a complete model involves characteristics of external and internal mass transfer, phase equilibrium, and flow pattern, the number of its parameters is too high to adjust all of them according to experimental extraction curves. As many parameters as possible should be fixed using additional information, e.g. the correlations published for external mass transfer coefficients, and the number of adjusted parameters should be minimized.

CHARACTERISTIC TIMES

The solvent has to penetrate into the particle and dissolve the extract, which then diffuses to the particle surface and further to bulk fluid phase, where its concentration is limited by equilibrium condition, and by convection it is removed from the extraction bed. To characterise the times necessary for each step separately, the rates of all other steps in mathematical model are assumed to be infinitely high. The following results are obtained.

Washing out

When all extract present in the extractor dissolves in the solvent already during the static extraction, the initial concentrations are:

$$ x_0 = 0, y_0 = x_u \frac{(1-\varepsilon)\rho_s}{\varepsilon \rho_f} = \frac{x_u}{\gamma} \quad (7) $$

A region of zero fluid phase concentration appears at the solvent inlet after the solvent starts flowing through extraction bed and extends with the solvent flow until the bed is emptied at the time equal to residence time, t_r, when $q = \gamma$ (Fig. 2).

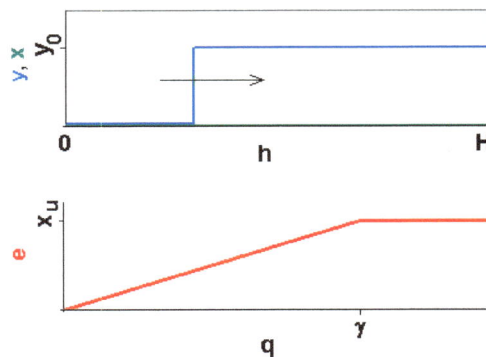

Figure 2: Concentration profiles and extraction curve for washing out.

Equilibrium-Controlled Extraction

On the assumption that equilibrium is established during the static extraction and the dynamic extraction takes place with the rate equal to the initial rate, the time necessary to remove all extract from the extraction bed minus the time necessary for washing out is:

$$t_{eq} = \frac{x_0}{q'y^*(x_0)} = \frac{x_0}{y^*(x_0)\gamma} t_r \qquad (8)$$

At this time, $q = x_0/y^*(x_0)$. Relating t_{eq} to t_r, the dimensionless time of equilibrium extraction is obtained:

$$\frac{t_{eq}}{t_r} = \frac{x_0}{y^*(x_0)\gamma} = \frac{1}{\Gamma} = \Theta_{eq} \qquad (9)$$

The corresponding concentration profiles and extraction curve are shown in Fig. **3**.

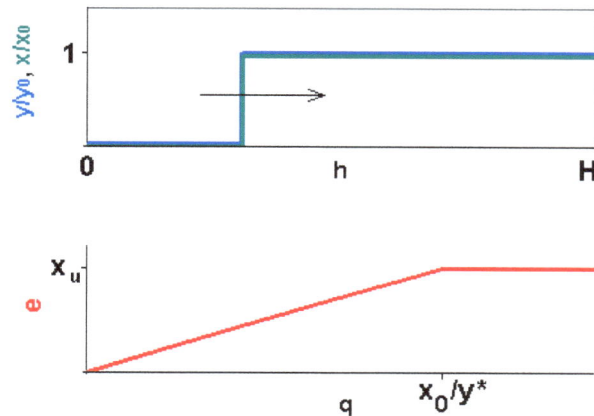

Figure 3: Concentration profiles and extraction curve for equilibrium-controlled extraction.

Internal Diffusion

When eqs. (3) and (5) are applied with $x^+ = 0$ and $x(t=0) = x_u$, the resulting extract concentration in particles and extraction yield are:

$$x = x_u \exp\left(-\frac{t}{t_i}\right), e = x_u\left[1 - \exp\left(-\frac{t}{t_i}\right)\right] \quad (10)$$

with time constant

$$t_i = \frac{1-\varepsilon}{k_s a_0} = \frac{\lambda}{k_s}. \qquad (11)$$

where λ is the characteristic particle dimension equal to its volume divided by its surface. When the solution of eq. (5a) is simplified assuming a parabolic concentration profile inside the spherical particle, eq. (10) applies, too, and its time constant is:

$$t_i = \frac{R^2}{15 D_{ef}} \qquad (12)$$

(see [4], [5]).

The difference between the extraction yield calculated according to eqs. (10), (12) and the exact solution of eqs. (3) and (5a), which represent the hot-ball model [6], is indicated in Fig. **4**.

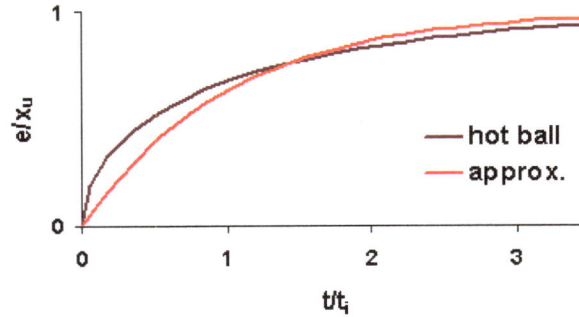

Figure 4: Internal diffusion-controlled extraction from spherical particles: hot-ball model and approximate solution given by eq. (10).

Similarly to Θ_{eq}, a dimensionless internal mass transfer resistance is introduced [7] as:

$$\Theta_i = \frac{t_i}{t_r} \qquad (13)$$

External Mass Transfer

In the case of extraction controlled solely by external mass transfer, the fluid phase concentration and the extraction yield are given by an equation analogous to eq. (10):

$$x = x_u \exp\left(-\frac{t}{t_e}\right), e = x_u\left[1-\exp\left(-\frac{t}{t_e}\right)\right] \qquad (14)$$

where the time constant and the dimensionless external mass transfer resistance are:

$$t_e = \frac{\varepsilon}{k_f a_0}, \Theta_e = \frac{t_e}{t_r} \qquad (15)$$

Time dependence of fluid and solid phase concentrations and extraction curve for both external and internal mass transfer is shown in Fig. **5**.

To sum up, the processes of equilibrium extraction and washing out are characterised by sharp concentration profiles moving in the direction of solvent flow, their extraction curves are straight lines, and their yields are directly proportional to solvent-to-feed ratio and do not depend on extraction time. On the opposite, the concentration profiles for the extraction controlled by internal and/or external mass transfer are flat, the extraction curves follow an exponential function of time and the extraction rate is independent of the solvent flow rate.

When the extraction consists of several subsequent steps and the characteristic time of one step is much larger than the others, the process is controlled by this step and the other steps can be neglected in the model. Comparing several experimental extraction curves measured at different specific flow rates, extraction periods controlled by one of these extraction steps can often be revealed and the model can be simplified for given period. The whole extraction process from the beginning to the end, however, is only rarely controlled by one extraction step. Such equilibrium-controlled extraction of essential oil from peppermint leaves was described by Goto et al. [8], and a solely internal mass transfer-controlled extraction of essential oils from plant particles was examined by Catchpole et al. [5] and Reverchon et al. [9], [10].

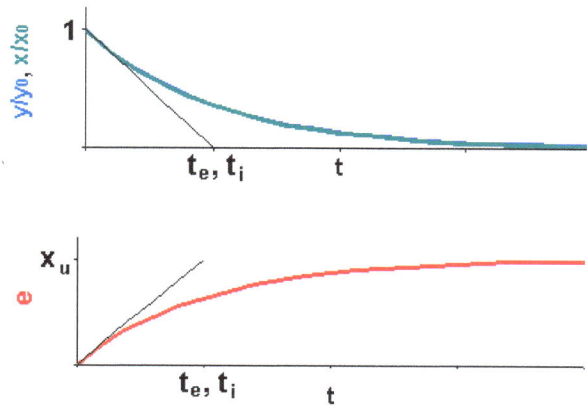

Figure 5: Concentration profiles and extraction curve for mass transfer-controlled extraction: time constant is t_e for external mass transfer or t_i for internal mass transfer.

EXTRACTION STEPS

Solubility and Phase Equilibrium

The equilibrium concentration of extract in supercritical solvent is either equal to its solubility or lower than the solubility, when the extract is bound to matrix. In both cases the equilibrium concentration strongly depends on extraction pressure and temperature.

Different scientific disciplines use different units to express the content of solute in the mixture. Thus, mole fractions are used in thermodynamic calculations, for diffusion and mass transfer generally the solute content is expressed as volumetric concentration, while mass fractions or mass ratios are used with advantage when the density of solution strongly varies like between the extractor and separator in the equipment for supercritical fluid extraction. The conversion from the volume-related units, c, c_s and $<c_s>$, in which the equilibrium relationships were originally formulated, to the mass-related units, x and y, is based on the assumption of constant density of fluid phase (which is regarded equal to the density of pure solvent, ρ_f, due to usually low solubility of extract in the solvent) and on the assumption of constant volume of the plant particles with initial density ρ_s, regardless of diminishing extract in them:

$$x = \frac{\langle c_s \rangle}{\rho_s}, y = \frac{c}{\rho_f} \qquad (16)$$

The density of supercritical CO_2 can be read from the tables or calculated using Bender equation of state with 21 coefficients [11] or the equation of state derived by Altunin and Gadetskii [12].

Solubilities of pure substances in supercritical solvents have to be determined experimentally in dependence on pressure and temperature. Parameters of a cubic equation of state of the mixture can be evaluated using these experimental data, provided the critical properties of the mixture constituents are known. The critical properties of many plant components, however, must be estimated because these substances decompose at temperatures far below their hypothetical critical temperature. The semi-empirical correlation of solubility with temperature and solvent density published by Chrastil [13] offers the possibility to interpolate the experimental solubility data:

$$y_s = \rho_f^{k-1} \exp\left(\frac{a}{T} + b\right) \quad (17)$$

The Chrastil equation uses adjustable coefficients a, b, k, where k is the average number of solvent molecules associated in the solution with one molecule of extract. A modification of eq. (17) was derived by del Valle and Aguilera [14] for common vegetable oils C54 (composed of fatty acid esters where fatty acids with 18 carbons in molecule prevail):

$$y_s = \rho_f{}^{9.724} \exp\left(-33.7178 - \frac{18708}{T} + \frac{2186840}{T^2}\right) \qquad (18)$$

The correlation is valid in a relatively wide range of pressures and temperatures

Fluid phase concentrations equal to extract solubility in the solvent are observed particularly in supercritical extraction of oils from seeds containing large amount of extract, tens of percent. Most of other substances extracted from plants occur in concentration of a few percent or even less and usually are bound to matrix. This becomes evident from their equilibrium relationship: as the solid phase concentration diminishes during the extraction, the equilibrium fluid phase concentration is decreasing, too. The extract may be adsorbed on solid matrix [8] or absorbed in a liquid contained in the plant [15]. Description of extract-matrix interaction by linear equilibrium relationship with partition coefficient K is mathematically simple and most frequent in the literature on SFE ([16], [8], [4], [17]):

$$y^* = Kx^*, c^* = K_v c_s{}^*, K = K_v \frac{\rho_s}{\rho_f} \qquad (19)$$

When the model for supercritical fluid extraction is simplified assuming a parabolic concentration profile in particles, eq. (19) is used to introduce linear driving force, and the surface concentrations are eliminated from the expression for mass transfer rate:

$$j = \frac{k_f a_0 \rho_f}{1 + \Gamma\, t_i/t_e}(Kx - y) = k a_0 \rho_f (Kx - y) \qquad (4a)$$

The modified models with parabolic concentration profile and linear driving force were published by Peker et al. [16] and Goto et al. [18], who corrected a typographical error found in [16].

In terms of mass transfer coefficients, the combined mass transfer coefficient is:

$$k = \frac{k_f}{1 + K_v k_f/k_s} \qquad (20)$$

As a function of Biot number it is for a spherical particle:

$$k = \frac{5 k_f}{5 + K_v Bi} \quad \text{where } Bi = \frac{k_f R}{D_{ef}} \qquad (21)$$

(see eqs. (11), (12)). Other relationships used in the SFE models for extract interaction with plant matrix are Langmuir adsorption isotherm [3], [19], Freundlich adsorption isotherm [20], and other adsorption isotherms [21]. Perrut et al. [22] observed during the extraction of oil from sunflower seed a composed equilibrium relationship, shifting near a certain critical solid phase concentration from the solubility to the linear equilibrium, and approximated it as follows:

$$y^* = y_s \text{ for } x \geq x_t,\ y^* = Kx \text{ for } x < x_t,\ Kx_t < y_s \qquad (22)$$

The relationship, depicted in Fig. **6**, has proved to be an efficient tool in SFE [23].

Goto et al. [24] applied in SFE modelling the BET isotherm, a three-parametric equation frequently used in adsorption/desorption theory. This relationship, similarly to eq. (22), combines the extract-matrix interaction for low solid phase concentration and solubility as asymptotic value for high extract concentration in plant. The transition from one to the other relation is, however, not as fast as many experimental data on SFE indicate.

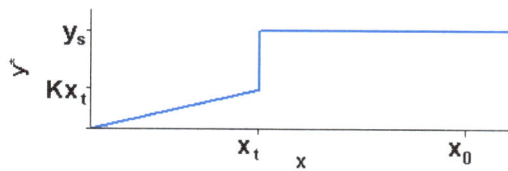

Figure 6: Equilibrium relationship [22] for seed oil extracted with supercritical CO_2.

External Mass Transfer

The properties of supercritical fluids are strongly dependent on pressure and temperature and generally most of them are between those of liquids and gases. It is so also for dynamic viscosity and for density, which is, however, usually adjusted close to density of liquids in order to obtain a sufficient solvent power. Kinematic viscosity as the dynamic viscosity-to-density ratio is therefore very low and binary diffusion coefficients of extracted substances in supercritical fluids as well as external mass transfer coefficients, k_f, are high. The k_f values also increase with increasing solvent velocity, and their order of magnitude is at usual conditions of SFE with carbon dioxide 10^{-6} or 10^{-5} m/s [25]. As the order of magnitude of the specific surface of particles in extraction bed is usually 10^3 m^2/m^3, the time constant of external mass transfer t_e (see eq. (15)) is typically expressed in tens or hundreds of seconds and thus it is usually lower than t_i, t_{eq} and also t_r. It can be determined experimentally comparing the slopes of initial straight parts of two extraction curves measured at different residence times, once at a high residence time when the solution is saturated and once at a low residence time when the effect of t_e on the slope of extraction curve becomes evident. Brunner [26] illustrated on experiments with SFE of oil from crushed seeds that the slope of extraction curve $e(q)$ in its initial straight part corresponding to the extraction from particle surface is:

$$y(H,t) = y_s\left[1 - \exp\left(-\frac{1}{\Theta_e}\right)\right] \qquad (23)$$

As the effect of external mass transfer of extraction curve is relatively small, the k_f value to be inserted into mathematical models for SFE is usually not measured but estimated from literature correlations derived for the flow in packed bed. The correlations, given in terms of dimensionless numbers Sh = Sh(Re, Sc), were reviewed recently by del Valle and de la Fuente [1]. When the term of external mass transfer resistance can be neglected in comparison with internal mass transfer resistance, the only mass transfer coefficient used in the model is k_s [4].

Internal Mass Transfer

The internal mass transfer resistance depends on many factors: what plant and what part of the plant (leaves, flowers, fruit, seed, root etc.) is extracted, where the extract is located in the material and what was the pretreatment of the material (drying, soaking with a liquid, different procedures of mechanical disintegration, opening the cavities containing the extract by a sudden decrease of pressure after pressurisation, and others). When non-polar and low-polar substances are extracted, the plant is usually dried as larger amounts of water would hinder the access of supercritical CO_2 into particles. The moisture of dry plants is usually slightly below 10 %, and during the SFE further decreases as water is co-extrated: the water solubility in supercritical CO_2 is approximately 1.5 mg/g at 25 °C, 3 mg/g at 50 °C and 5 mg/g at 75 °C [27]. The permeability of cell membranes changes with water content; they become impermeable when there is not enough water in the plant [28].The extremely low values of effective diffusion coefficient, observed frequently in SFE, can be explained by low content of water in over-dried plants. On the other hand, the particles soaked with water, which can be applied in SFE of polar compounds as alkaloids, are well permeable.

Plant particles are often described as porous bodies with the pores filled with solution of extract in the solvent; the extract diffuses through the pores to particle surface. The internal porosity is measured independently from SFE experiments, at ambient pressure. The effective diffusion coefficient is then estimated from the binary diffusion coefficient [1], [29] as:

$$D_{ef} = D_{12}\frac{\beta}{\tau} \qquad (24)$$

or even simpler, when the tortuosity is estimated as the inverse value of particle porosity [8], as:

$$D_{ef} = D_{12}\beta^2 \quad \text{(24a)}$$

Flow Pattern

Eq. (2) is written for the plug flow pattern, where the solvent flows in axial direction and its velocity is of the same value in the whole extractor. In reality, axial dispersion exists in the flow through a packed bed due to molecular diffusion and flow irregularities, and the mass balance equation should therefore include an axial dispersion term:

$$\varepsilon\rho_f\left(\frac{\partial y}{\partial t} + u\frac{\partial y}{\partial h} - D_{ax}\frac{\partial^2 y}{\partial h^2}\right) = J, \frac{u}{\varepsilon}y - D_{ax}\frac{\partial y}{\partial h} = 0 \text{ for } h = 0, \frac{\partial y}{\partial h} = 0 \text{ for } h = H \quad \text{(2a)}$$

with D_{ax}, the axial dispersion coefficient ([30]-[32]). The values of D_{ax} in SFE models are usually estimated from correlations of Peclet number, e.g. the correlation published by Tan and Liou [33]. Many researchers observed, however, that the term for axial dispersion with D_{ax} values estimated this way had negligible or very small effect on the calculated extraction yield ([17], [34], [35]) and therefore eq. (2) is used frequently in the models instead of eq. (2a).

For a short extraction bed a lumped parameter model (model of differential extractor) is applied ([16], [8]). The fluid phase mass balance equation is then an ordinary differential equation identical with that for ideal mixer:

$$\rho_f\varepsilon\left(\frac{dy}{dt} + \frac{y}{t_r}\right) = J, \ y(t = 0) = y_0 \quad \text{(2b)}$$

When eq. (2b) is combined with eqs. (1) and (3), mass transfer resistance is neglected and linear equilibrium according to eq. (19) is assumed, the model for equilibrium extraction yields an extraction curve which shape is identical with that shown in Fig. **5** but the argument of the exponential function is now proportional to the solvent-to-feed ratio, not to the extraction time. Thus, the exponential shape of extraction curve does not always indicate a mass transfer controlled extraction; to distinguish between the equilibrium extraction and the mass transfer controlled extraction, experiments at different residence times must be conducted and compared.

Comparing the rate of SFE with the solvent flow from extractor bottom upwards and with the flow in the opposite direction, the extraction with the flow to the bottom was sometimes found faster ([36], [37]), and this effect was more pronounced at low interstitial velocities [38]. The effect is connected with natural convection that easily develops in supercritical fluids due to their low kinematic viscosity. The loaded solvent is usually heavier than pure one and flows faster downwards. It is not yet clear whether the natural convection takes place on micro scale, increasing the external mass transfer coefficient in gravity-assisted flow and decreasing it in gravity-opposed flow, as suggested by Recasens and co-workers ([39], [40]) or whether it acts on a larger scale, changing flow pattern in the extractor. In any case, the inhomogeneity of solvent flow resulting from the inhomogeneity of extraction bed porosity is more pronounced at low velocities when the flow direction is upwards (Dams [38], Sovova et al. [41]). The SFE retarded by natural convection was simulated dividing the flow in the extractor into parallel flows of different velocities and thus different outlet concentrations [39]. The model was and later applied to simulate the scale-up effect [34].

SFE FROM WELL PERMEABLE PARTICLES

Using relationships for equilibrium concentration y*, external and internal mass transfer parameters, and flow pattern, the SFE models define all extraction steps – dissolving the extract in the solvent, its diffusion to particle surface, and its transfer in the solvent phase out of the extraction bed. According to underlying assumptions on the structure of plant particles and on the initial extract location, diffusion models, desorption models, and shrinking core models can be distinguished. Peker et al. [16] derived a model for SFE of caffeine from water-soaked coffee beans. They described the beans as porous spherical particles of specified radius and porosity, whose pores are filled with water. A linear adsorption equilibrium characterised by a partition coefficient is assumed to be established on the pore walls where the extract desorbs from solid matrix into water. The diffusion in the pores is characterised by effective diffusion coefficient. The equilibrium at particle surface is given by a linear relationship where another partition coefficient characterises the partitioning of caffeine between supercritical carbon dioxide and water. Finally, to describe the extract diffusion through boundary layer to bulk fluid, the external mass transfer coefficient is used. This model combines a desorption model for desorption at the pore walls and a diffusion model with equilibrium on particle surface. A lumped parameter model was used, adequate for the small extractor of 1.27 cm height and 1.73 cm inner diameter, and analytical solution of model equations with two time constants was obtained when a parabolic concentration profile in particles leading to application of linear driving force was assumed.

Diffusion Models

These models describe the internal diffusion of extract to particle surface where equilibrium is established, and its external diffusion to bulk fluid. The above mentioned model for the extraction of caffeine [16] was simplified by its authors to a diffusional model, assuming that all coffeine in the beans is dissolved in water filling the pores. The partition coefficient for caffeine between water in particle pores and supecritical carbon model parameter adjusted according to experimental extraction curves; the k_f value was computed with the Wakao and Kaguei correlation [42] and D_{ef} was taken from the literature.

Catchpole et al. [5] modified the diffusion model with linear equilibrium and lumped parameters for plug flow pattern. The assumption of parabolic concentration profiles in particles was applied, too, in order to introduce linear driving force and simplify the set of model equations. For a special case of internal diffusion-controlled extraction the model was reduced to eq. (10) with characteristic times defined for a sphere, a cylinder and a slab. To determine D_{ef}, eq. (10) was compared with experimental data on the SFE of oleoresin from celery, sage and coriander (Table 1). The complete model equations were used to calculate the yield of oil in the SFE from coriander seeds. This process was not only internal diffusion dependent but also, at least for the smaller particles, equilibrium dependent, which was evident from the sensitivity of extraction curve to the changes in flow pattern, introduced by changing the extractor geometry and the solvent flow direction.

Goodarznia and Ekani [31] derived a diffusion model with axial dispersion in fluid phase and with linear equilibrium at the surface of spherical particles, described the technique of its numerical solution, and applied it to literature data on SFE of essential oils.

Reverchon [4] neglected the external mass transfer resistance in the diffusion model for SFE of essential oil from sage leaves, assumed a plug flow pattern, and used the approximate relationship for characteristic internal diffusion time:

$$t_i = \mu \frac{\lambda^2}{D_{ef}} \qquad (12a)$$

where μ is equal to 3/5 for spheres, 1/2 for cylinders and 1/3 for slabs. When applied to experiments with SFE from particles of different sizes, the model for spherical particles overestimated the effect of particle size. On the other hand, when a more realistic assumption of particles as slabs of a constant thickness was made, the prediction of the effect of particle size on the extraction rate was very good.

Poletto and Reverchon [7] performed a parametric analysis of the diffusion model with plug flow pattern and with linear equilibrium at particle surface. They assumed the existence of either internal or external mass transfer resistance but their analysis can easily be modified for a model with total mass transfer resistance $\Theta = \Gamma \Theta_i + \Theta_e. = t_i/t_{eq} + t_e/t_r$, compatible with eq. (4a). Three regions of Θ values were distinguished. For $\Theta < 0.02$, the model for equilibrium-controlled extraction is recommended (Fig. **2**). For $\Theta > 2$, the concentration profiles in extraction bed are flat and a lumped parameter model can be applied. For Θ values between these limits, equations of the complete model should be integrated numerically.

A further analysis of the diffusion model with linear equilibrium at particle surface and with plug flow was made for spherical particles by del Valle et al. [17]. The model equations were integrated numerically using a fourth-order Runge-Kutta method. The effects of both total mass transfer resistance and individual resistances were examined. The authors recommended to compare the results of model calculations with experimental data not only in terms of extraction curves but also in terms of residual solid phase concentration profiles $x(h)$ measured after the extraction was stopped early enough to leave approximately half of the extract in the particles; a better distinction between different models is then possible. The modified model equations, where either internal or external mass transfer resistance was neglected, were also solved numerically. When the model without external mass transfer resistance was applied on the results of SFE of volatile oil from basil leaves [9], practically identical value of D_{ef} (see Table 1) was obtained as the value given in the original paper on the basis of a modified hot-ball model. It is a confirmation of the fact that in the case of low permeable particles, when the time constant of internal diffusion largely prevails over the characteristic constants of other extraction steps, simple models resulting in the extraction curves shown in Fig. **4** are sufficient.

Desorption Models

In these models the particles are porous bodies. The extract is desorbed from pore walls into the solvent filling the pores and diffuses to particle surface from where it is transferred to bulk fluid. Thus, the extract concentrations in the pores and in the boundary layer are equal at particle surface ($K_v = 1$). Goto et al. [8] reduced the desorption-diffusion-partitioning model with lumped parameters [16] to a desorption model and applied its simplified version with analytical solution to the SFE of essential oil from peppermint leaves. The extractor dimensions were 5.0 cm height and 2.3 cm inner diameter. The adsorption equilibrium constant was adjusted according to experimental data, the value of D_{ef} was calculated according to eq. (24a) and k_f was estimated from the Wakao and Kaguei (1985) correlation [42]. The extraction was found to be equilibrium-controlled; the resistances Θ_e and Θ_i were small compared to Θ_{eq}.

A desorption model for the flow with axial dispersion and with the BET adsorption isotherm was published by Goto et al. [24]. The observed difference in the extraction behaviour of essential oil and cuticular wax extracted simultaneously from peppermint leaves was explained in terms of their different BET equilibrium constants: the extraction of strongly adsorbed essential oil was found to be equilibrium-controlled and the extraction of weakly adsorbed wax was mass transfer controlled.

Shrinking Core Models

Application of these extraction models is restricted to porous spherical particles. The pores in the core, the central part of the particle, are completely filled with extract. The core radius is initially equal to the radius of the particle; as the extract dissolves in the solvent and the extraction proceeds, the core shrinks. The interface is located on the core surface and the fluid phase equilibrium concentration is equal to the solubility of extract in the solvent, y_s. The internal mass transfer resistance acts outside the core in the pores filled with the solution; the length of the diffusion path increases as the core shrinks from zero value at $t = 0$. Parametric analysis of shrinking core model with axial dispersion was performed by Goto et al. [30]. One of the most important parameters was $a = 15\Theta_i$. For $a = 10$, the process was not far from the equilibrium-controlled extraction, with steep concentration profiles in both phases and with an initial constant extraction rate period evident on extraction curve. For $a = 50$ and $a = 100$, the concentration profiles were rather flat and the local mass transfer rates were similar in the whole extraction bed. The effect of axial dispersion is important only at small values of a. Even then it becomes insignificant when Peclet number is larger than 100. Similarly to the internal mass transfer resistance, a high external mass transfer resistance also flattens the concentration profiles. The model was applied to experimental data on SFE of oil from pre-pressed seeds published by Brunner [26]. The k_f value was calculated from the Wakao and Kaguei correlation [42]. Peclet number was estimated to 50, it is with practically no influence of axial dispersion on extraction curves, and D_{ef} as the most important parameter was obtained by fitting the calculated results to experimental data (Table 1).

The shrinking core models are adequate when the solute content in the plant material is large, like in the case of oil in seeds, so that it can completely fill the particle pores [1].

Table 1: Effective internal diffusion coefficients, D_{ef}, evaluated using the models for well permeable particles and the models for internal diffusion controlled SFE.

Extract	Matrix	D_{ef}, m^2/s	References
volatile oil[a]	leaves	$(1-15)\ 10^{-9}$	[8]
caffeine[a]	water-soaked beans	$(1-3)10^{-10}$	[16]
oil[a]	pre-pressed seed	$(0.7-1.5)10^{-10}$	[26], [29]
oil[a]	seed	$2.6\ 10^{-11}$	[5]
volatile oil[b]	aerial parts, seed	$(1-5)\ 10^{-12}$	[5]
volatile oil[a]	leaves	$6\ 10^{-13}$	[4]
volatile oil[b]	leaves	$(1-2)\ 10^{-13}$	[9], [17]

[a]model for well permeable particle

[b]model for internal diffusion-controlled SFE

SFE FROM PARTICLES WITH BROKEN AND INTACT CELLS

A relatively sharp transition from the initial straight line corresponding to constant extraction rate to a curved section corresponding to a slower extraction was observed on extraction curves in SFE, particularly when oil was extracted from oilseed particles. The first period was related to the extraction of oil located on particle surface, which was released from the seeds by mechanical treatment [26]. The extraction is thus independent of internal mass transfer and its rate is according to eq. (23) determined by extract solubility and dimensionless external mass transfer resistance. When $\Theta < 0.2$ and the extract does not interact with matrix, the solution at the extractor outlet is practically saturated.

The final part of extraction curve, on the other hand, corresponds to the internal diffusion controlled extraction from intact cells. The extraction yield in this period therefore follows a modified eq. (10):

$$e = x_u - C_1 \exp\left(-\frac{t}{t_i} \right) \quad (10a)$$

Eq. (10a) was fitted to final parts of experimental extraction curves of different plants extracted with liquid carbon dioxide in order to to evaluate the internal mass transfer coefficients [43] or to estimate the overall content of extract in plant samples, x_u, for the purpose of sample analysis [44].

A combination of these two equations for the first and second extraction periods was proposed by Goodrum et al. [45] for SFE of peanut oil and by Yoo and Hong [46] for the extraction of oilseeds generally. A model based on mass balance equations for plug flow where the term for local mass transfer switches from free dissolution to a slower extraction of the extract interacting with matrix when the solid phase concentration decreases to a certain value was adapted from a model for drying by Lack under supervision of R. Marr [47]. The model was further modified by Sovova [48] for the extraction of low soluble extracts like oil from seed, controlled first by external and then by internal mass transfer, and its approximate solution was adopted from [47]. An important improvement of the model was made in the group of E. Reverchon where separate mass balances were written for the easily accessible extract in broken cells on particle surface and for the extract closed in intact cells ([49], [35]). The equilibrium fluid phase concentration of oil on particle surface was equal to its solubility, while the equilibrium of oil from intact cells was given by the linear relationship.

All models based on the concept of broken and intact cells contain a parameter concerning the initial distribution of extract between the broken and intact cells. It can be e.g. the fraction of extract in broken cells, ranging from 0 to 1. Usually it is adjusted comparing the experimental extraction curves with calculated ones. Reverchon and co-workers tried to determine it independently analysing images of particle surface obtained by scanning electron microscope, estimating the depth of the layer of broken cells on particle surface and relating its volume to the volume of whole particle. It seems, however, that the real fraction of extract in broken cells is higher than according to this method, it means, some cells in lower layers are broken, too.

The concept of separate mass balances for broken and intact cells was applied to develop a more general model where different equilibrium relationships may be included as necessary and different degrees of axial mixing are simulated, adjusting the number of mixers into which the extractor is divided [23]. A relationship between the complete model and its simplified version is described in the paper, too. A model with broken and intact cells and with a series of mixers was used already ten years earlier to model both small-scale and large-scale supercritical fluid extraction from plants [50]. A further development of the BIC models was presented by Zizovic and co-workers particularly for SFE of essential oils. They took into account the structure of particles and the location of extract in different families of plants and modelled on microscale the process of opening of essential oil-containing glandular trichomes on leaf surface under supercritical CO_2 pressure [51] and the diffusion in secretory ducts [52]. These models were recently summarised and further improved [53].

SCALE-UP

One of the main tasks of mathematical modelling of SFE is to enable extrapolation from pilot plant to industrial scale extraction. A very simple method of the extrapolation is to keep both specific flow rate and extraction time in the larger equipment equal to those in the smaller one so that the same extraction yield should be achieved regardless of whether the process is equilibrium- or mass transfer-controlled [50]. Using the above discussed models with the mass transfer and equilibrium parameters based on experimental data measured in a pilot plant, however, it is not difficult to calculate extraction curves for any feed size, any solvent flow rate, and any extraction time, regardless of differences in extraction time and solvent-to feed ratio.

Experimental data illustrating the effects of scale-up on extraction yield can be found in the literature; usually they concern the transition from laboratory equipment to pilot plant. The scale-up for SFE of evening primrose oil from pilot plant with an extractor of 20 L volume to industrial equipment with extractor volume 0.2 m^3 was described by Eggers and Sievers [54]. In the first extraction period, dependent on the external mass transfer, the extraction yield in the larger extractor was even slightly higher than in pilot extractor. The reason is that when the specific flow rate was kept constant, the flow velocity was higher in the larger extractor of similar height-to-diameter ratio, therefore also the external mass transfer coefficient was higher and the dimensionless external mass transfer resistance Θ_e was lower.

In most cases, however, the performance of the larger extractor is found to be lower than the predictions based on pilot plant data indicate. The main reason behind it is a change in the solvent flow pattern. The extraction bed in the larger extractor is usually less homogeneous than the bed in a smaller extractor and thus the solvent flow distribution is not uniform. The effect of sticking together of particles containing on their surface liquid extract is also more pronounced when the height of extraction bed and thus also the weight acting on lower layers of particles is larger. When any flow irregularities and, as a consequence, also differences in local mass transfer rate and in concentrations and fluid phase densities develop, they may be stabilised by natural convection.

Such unfavourable deviations from plug flow should be taken into account in the scale-up procedure, and *vice versa*, when the difference between the real extraction yield in the larger equipment and its prediction based on pilot data is too large, measures should be taken to better distribute the solvent flow, using a properly designed distributor, a better procedure of filling the extractor with particles, mixing the sticky particles with inert material, changing the particle size, etc. Particles of mean size lower than 0.4 mm should not be loaded into a larger extractor because channelling often occurs in such extraction beds: extremely small particles are easily pressed to form a dense impermeable layer where only a few channels are formed. The solvent escapes through them without any sufficient contact with solid phase and the extraction is therefore heavily retarded. An elegant solution to this problem is pelletisation of vegetable material after its milling to powder. The internal diffusion is then fast due broken cell walls but hydrodynamic resistance of the pellets is small and thus there is no danger of channelling.

The effect of scale-up from a laboratory extractor (feed 26 g of hiprose seeds) to a pilot plant with CO$_2$ recycle (feed 800 g of seed) was studied and the experimental extraction curves were modelled by del Valle et al. [34]. Three hypothesis on the extraction retardation observed in the larger extractor were tested: (i) the separation of extract from solvent in the separator behind the extractor is not complete and thus a part of the extracted oil is recycled, (ii) the axial dispersion is increased in the larger extractor, (iii) there are two regions of different solvent velocity in the extractor. The model based on the third hypothesis enabled a close simulation of experimental extraction curves.

Another example of scale-up was published by Berna et al. [55] who extracted essential oil from orange peels in a laboratory extractor (0.36 L) and in a pilot plant (5.18 L) at pressure of 20 MPa and temperature of 40 °C. The essential oil is completely miscible with CO$_2$ under these conditions. Two cultivars were extracted; naveline cultivar contained 12.6 wt. % essential oil and satsuma cultivar contained 5.8 wt. %. The extraction curves consist of three parts: the washing-out period when the solution of essential oil dissolved in CO$_2$ during the pressurization is obtained, the linear equilibrium- and external mass transfer-controlled extraction period, when the essential oil is desorbed from plant matrix and thus its fluid phase equilibrium concentration is lower than in the first period, and finally the internal diffusion-controlled period. The particles of peels of satsuma cultivar were sticky and thus the flow was not regular in the larger extractor, though its inhomogeneity was reduced by addition of a layer of inert particles as solvent flow distributor at the bottom where the solvent entered the extraction. Except for the first extraction period, the solvent loading was lower in the larger extractor (Fig. **7**). Assuming equilibrium extraction in the smaller extractor in the second extraction period, the dimensionless external mass transfer resistance in the larger extractor can be estimated to $\Theta_e = 1.7$.

The naveline cultivar contained more essential oil and its particles were therefore even more aggregated. Besides, no measures were taken to improve the flow distribution in the extraction bed. As a result, the reduction in extraction rate in the larger extractor was more pronounced than in the case of the satsuma cultivar (Fig. **8**). Assuming equilibrium extraction in the smaller extractor, the dimensionless external mass transfer resistance in the larger extractor is estimated to $\Theta_e = 5.5$, an unusually high value in SFE.

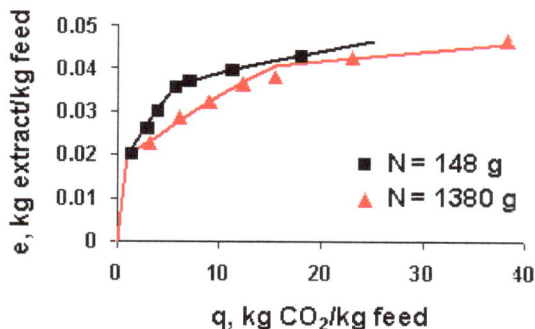

Figure 7: SFE of essential oil from orange peel (satsuma cultivar) [55]. Flow distributor was used in the larger equipment to suppress flow inhomogeneities.

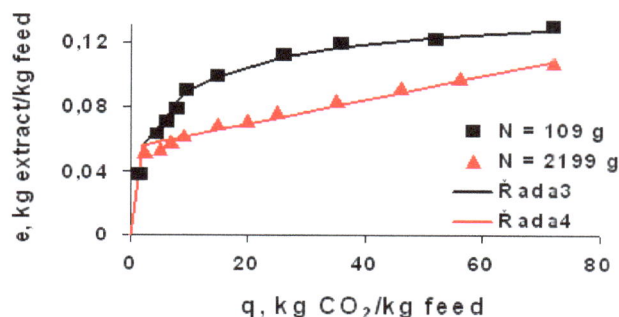

Figure 8: SFE of essential oil from orange peel (naveline cultivar) [55]. No flow distributor was used.

CONCLUSIONS

Different mathematical models have been published for supercritical fluid extraction of natural products from plant materials. To choose the proper model, it is important to compare the estimates of time constants of external and internal mass transfer and the characteristic times of equilibrium extraction and washing out. Pretreatment of dry plants by mechanical disintegration (grinding, milling, cutting, chopping, pressing etc.) or other methods, like a rapid depressurisation, has great effect on extraction kinetics as it breaks cell walls, improves the matrix permeability, shortens diffusion paths and increases surface area. Models for well permeable particles should be used when the time constant of internal diffusion is comparable with characteristic time of equilibrium extraction. In other cases, when a non-negligible part of extract remains closed in intact cells, the models distinguishing between the extraction from broken and intact cells should be applied. Deviations of the solvent flow pattern from plug flow, which can be significant particularly in larger extractors, result in reduction of extraction rate and should be therefore minimised by improving the flow distribution.

ACKNOWLEDGEMENTS

The author thanks the Grant Agency of the Czech Republic for financial support (project No. 104/06/1174).

NOMENCLATURE

a_0 : specific surface area, m^2/m^3
Bi   : $(=k_f R/D_{ef})$ Biot number, -
c : fluid phase concentration, kg/m^3
c_s : solid phase concentration, kg/m^3

$<c_s>$	:	average concentration in particle, kg/m^3
d_p	:	particle equivalent diameter, m
D_{12}	:	binary effective diffusion coefficient of extract in the solvent, m^2/s
D_{ax}	:	effective diffusion coefficient, m^2/s
D_{ef}	:	effective diffusion coefficient, m^2/s
e	:	(= E/N) extraction yield, kg/kg
E	:	extract, kg
h	:	axial coordinate, m
H	:	height of extraction bed, m
j	:	mass transfer rate, kg/m^3 s
k	:	combined mass transfer coefficient, m/s
k_f	:	external mass transfer coefficient, m/s
k_s	:	internal mass transfer coefficient, m/s
K	:	(=$K_V \rho_s / \rho_f$) partition coefficient, (kg/kg)/(kg/ kg)
K_V	:	partition coefficient, (kg/m^3)/(kg/m^3)
N	:	feed of plant material, kg
Pe	:	(=Hu/D_{ax})Peclet number
q	:	(=Q/N) solvent-to-feed, kg/kg
q'	:	(=Q'/N) specific flow rate, kg/kg s
Q	:	(=$Q't$) solvent passed through extractor, kg
Q'	:	flow rate, kg/s
r	:	radial coordinate, m
R	:	particle radius, m
Re	:	(=$u \varepsilon d_p \rho_f / \mu$) Reynolds number
Sc	:	(=$\mu / \rho_f D_{12}$) Schmidt number
Sh	:	(=$k_f / d_p D_{12}$) Sherwood number
t	:	extraction time, s
t_e	:	(=$\varepsilon / (k_f a_0)$) time constant of external mass transfer, s
t_{eq}	:	(=$x_0 / (q' y_0^*)$) characteristic time of equilibrium extraction, s
t_i	:	time constant of internal diffusion, given by eqs. (11), (12), (12a), s
t_r	:	(= $u/H = \gamma / q'$) residence time, s
T	:	absolute temperature, K
u	:	interstitial velocity, m/s
x	:	extract content in solid phase, kg/kg
x^+	:	extract content in solid phase at particle surface, kg/kg
x^*	:	equilibrium extract content in solid phase, kg/kg
x_0	:	initial extract content in solid phase, kg/kg
x_t	:	transition concentration in eq. (22), kg/kg
x_u	:	extract in untreated solid phase, kg/kg
y	:	extract content in fluid phase, kg/(kg solvent)
y^+	:	extract content in fluid phase at particle surface, kg/(kg solvent)
y^*	:	equilibrium extract content in fluid phase, kg/(kg solvent)
y_0	:	initial extract content in fluid phase, kg/(kg solvent)
y_s	:	extract solubility, kg/(kg solvent)

Greek Letters

β	:	particle porosity, -
γ	:	(=$\varepsilon \rho_f / ((1-\varepsilon) \rho_s)$) fluid-to-solid ratio in extraction bed, kg/kg
Γ	:	(=$\gamma y_0^* / x_0$) equilibrium extract partition between fluid and solid phase, kg/kg
ε	:	void fraction in extraction bed, -
Θ	:	(=t/t_r) combined mass transfer resistance, -
Θ_e	:	(=t_e/t_r) external mass transfer resistance, -
Θ_{eq}	:	(=$t_{eq}/t_r = 1/\Gamma$) dimensionless equilibrium extraction time, -
Θ_i	:	(=t_i/t_r) internal mass transfer resistance, -
λ	:	characteristic particle dimension, m
μ	:	solvent viscosity, kg/m s

ρ_f : solvent density, kg/m^3
ρ_s : initial solid density, kg/m^3
τ : tortuosity, -

REFERENCES

[1]   del Valle, J.M.; de la Fuente, J.C. *Crit. Rev. Food Sci. Nutrition*, **2006**, 46, 131.
[2]   Reverchon, E. *J. Supercrit. Fluids*, **1997**, 10, 1.
[3]   Al-Jabari, M. *J. Sep. Sci.*, **2002**, 25, 477.
[4]   Reverchon, E. *AIChE J.*, **1996**, 42, 1765.
[5]   Catchpole, O.J.; Grey, J.B.; Smallfield, B.M. *J. Supercrit. Fluids*, **1996**, 9, 273.
[6]   Bartle, K.D.; Clifford, A.A.; Hawthorne, S.B.; Langenfeld, J.J.; Miller, D.J.; Robinson, R. *J. Supercrit. Fluids*, **1990**, 3, 143.
[7]   Poletto, M.; Reverchon, E. *Ind. Eng. Chem. Res.*, **1996**, 35, 3680.
[8]   Goto, M.; Sato, M.; Hirose, T. *J. Chem. Eng. Japan*, **1993**, 26, 401.
[9]   Reverchon, E.; Donsi, G.; Sesti Osseo, L. *Ind. Eng. Chem. Res.*, **1993**, 32, 2721.
[10]   Reverchon, E.; Sesti Osseo, L.; Gorgoglione, D. *J. Supercrit. Fluids*, **1994**, 7, 185.
[11]   Brunner, G. *Gas Extraction. An Introduction to Fundamentals of Supercritical Fluids and the Application to Separation Processes*; Springer: New York, USA, **1994**; pp. 15-16.
[12]   Angus, S.; Armstrong, B.; de Reuck, K. M. *International Thermodynamic Tables of Fluid State, Carbon Dioxide*; Pergamon Press: Oxford, UK, **1976**; pp. 37, 45-47.
[13]   Chrastil, J. *J. Phys. Chem.*, **1982**, 86, 3016.
[14]   del Valle, J.M.; Aguilera, J.M. *Ind. Eng. Chem. Res.*, **1988**, 27, 1551.
[15]   Sovova, H.; Stateva, R.P.; Galushko, A.A. *J. Supercrit. Fluids*, **2001**, 20, 113.
[16]   Peker, H.; Srinivasan, M.P.; Smith, J.M.; McCoy, B.J. *AIChE J.*, **1992**, 38, 761.
[17]   del Valle, J.M.; Napolitano, P.; Fuentes, N. *Ind. Eng. Chem. Res.*, **2000**, 39, 4720.
[18]   Goto, M.; Hirose, T.; McCoy, B.J. *J. Supercrit. Fluids*, **1994**, 7, 61.
[19]   Silva, C.F.; Mendes, M.F.; Pessoa, F.L.P.; Queiroz, E.M. *Brazil. J. Chem. Eng.*, **2008**, 25, 175.
[20]   Brunner, G. *Gas Extraction. An Introduction to Fundamentals of Supercritical Fluids and the Application to Separation Processes*; Springer: New York, USA, **1994**; pp. 224-225.
[21]   Salimi, A.; Fatemi, S.; Nei, H.Z.N.; Safaralie, A. Chem. Eng. Technol., **2008**, 31, 1470.
[22]   Perrut, M.; Clavier, J.Y.; Poletto, M.; Reverchon, E. Ind. Eng. Chem. Res., **1997**, 36, 430.
[23]   Sovova, H. *J. Supercrit. Fluids*, **2005**, 33, 35.
[24]   Goto, M.; Roy, B.C.; Kodama, A.; Hirose, T. *J. Chem. Eng. Jpn.*, **1998**, 31, 171.
[25]   Reverchon, E.; Marrone, C. *Chem. Eng. Sci.*, **1997**, 52, 3421.
[26]   Brunner, G. *Ber. Bunsenges. Phys. Chem.*, **1984**, 88, 887.
[27]   Wiebe, R.; Gaddy, V.L. *J. Am. Chem. Soc.*, **1941**, 63, 475.
[28]   Brunner, G. *Gas Extraction. An Introduction to Fundamentals of Supercritical Fluids and the Application to Separation Processes*; Springer: New York, USA, **1994**; pp. 183-185.
[29]   del Valle, J.M.; Germain, J.C.; Uquiche, E.; Zetzl, C.; Brunner, G. *J. Supercrit. Fluids*, **2006**, 37, 178.
[30]   Goto, M.; Roy, B.C.; Hirose, T. *J. Supercrit. Fluids*, **1996**, 9, 128.
[31]   Goodarznia, I.; Eikani, M.H. *Chem. Eng. Sci.*, **1998**, 53, 1387
[32]   Doker, O.; Salgin, U.; Sanal, I.; Mehmetoglu, U.; Calimli, A. *J. Supercrit. Fluids*, **2004**, 28, 11
[33]   Tan, C. S.; Liou, D. C. *Ind. Eng. Chem. Res.*, 1989, 28, 1246.
[34]   del Valle, J.M.; Rivera, O.; Mattea, M.; Ruetsch, L.; Daghero, J.; Flores, A. *J. Supercrit. Fluids*, **2004**, 31, 159.
[35]   Reverchon, E.; Marrone, C. *J. Supercrit. Fluids*, **2001**, 19, 161.
[36]   Beutler, H.J.; Gahrs, H.J.; Lenhard, U.; Lurken, F. *Chem. Ing. Tech.*, **1988**, 60, 773.
[37]   Barton, P.; Hughes, R.E.; Hussein, M.M. *J. Supercrit. Fluids*, **1992**, 5, 157.
[38]   Dams, A. *Chem. Ing. Tech.*, **1989**, 61, 712.
[39]   Stuber, F.; Vazquez, A.M.; Larrayoz, M.A.; Recasens, F. *Ind. Eng. Chem. Res.*, **1996**, 35, 3618.
[40]   Guardo, A.; Coussirat, M.; Recasens, F.; Larrayoz, M.A.; Escaler, X. *Chem. Eng. Sci.*, **2007**, 62, 5503.
[41]   Sovova, H.; Kucera, J.; Jez, J. *Chem. Eng. Sci.*, **1994**, 49, 415.
[42]   Wakao, N.; Kaguei, S. *Heat and Mass Transfer in Packed Beds*; Gordon and Breach: New York, USA, **1982**; p. 156.
[43]   Pekhov, A.V.; Goncharenko, G.K. *Maslo-Zhir. Prom.*, **1968**, 34(10), 26.
[44]   Dean, J.R.; Liu, B. Phytochem. Anal., **2000**, 11, 1.
[45]   Goodrum, J.W.; Kilgo, M.K.; Santerre, C.R. In: King, J.W.; List, G.R., Eds., *Supercritical Fluid Technology in Oil and Lipid Chemistry*; AOCS PressChampaign, Illinois, USA, **1996**, pp. 101-131.

[46] Yoo, K.P.; Hong, I.K. In: King, J.W.; List, G.R., Eds., *Supercritical Fluid Technology in Oil and Lipid Chemistry*; AOCS PressChampaign, Illinois, USA, **1996**, pp. 132-154.

[47] Lack, E.A., Ph.D.Thesis, TU Graz, Austria, **1985**.

[48] Sovova, H. *Chem. Eng. Sci.*, **1994**, 49, 409.

[49] Marrone, C.; Poletto, M.; Reverchon, E.; Stassi, A. *Chem. Eng. Sci.*, **1998**, 53, 3711.

[50] Clavier, J.Y.; Majewski, W; Perrut, M. Extrapolation from pilot plant to industrial scale SFE: a case study. In: Kikic, I; Alessi, P., Eds. Proceedings of the 3rd Italian Conference on Supercritical Fluids and their Application, **1995**: Grignano (Trieste), Italy: Universita di Trieste 1995; pp. 107-114.

[51] Zizovic, I.; Stamenic, M.; Orlovic, A.; Skala, D. *Chem. Eng. Sci.*, **2005**, 60, 6747.

[52] Zizovic, I.; Stamenic, M.; Ivanovic, J.; Orlovic, A.; Ristic, M.; Djordjevic, S.; Petrrovic, S.D.; Skala, D. *J. Supercrit. Fluids.*, **2007**, 43, 249.

[53] Stamenic, M.; Zizovic, I.; Orlovic, A Skala, D. *J. Supercrit. Fluids.*, **2008**, 46, 285.

[54] Eggers, R.; Sievers, U. In: Johnson, K.P.; Penninger, J.M.L., Eds., *Supercritical Fluid Science and Technology*; Am. Chem. Soc.: Washington D.C., USA, **1989**, p. 478.

[55] Berna, A.; Tarrega, A.; Blasco, M.; Subirats, S. *J. Supercrit. Fluids*, **2000**, 18, 227.

CHAPTER 10

Supercritical Fluid Processing in Food and Pharmaceutical Industries: Scale-Up Issues

Fabrice Leboeuf and Frantz Deschamps*

SEPAREX, 5 rue Jacques Monod, 54250 Champigneulles (France) Email: fdeschamps@separex.fr

Abstract: From the early 70s, supercritical fluid processing found numerous applications at industrial scale in the food industry through extraction and fractionation processes. In the same time, over the past two decades, a wide variety of supercritical fluid (SCF)-based processes dedicated to the design and engineering of particles were investigated mainly for applications in the pharmaceutical industry. Among these particle engineering processes, none of them reached commercial and full scale production yet in the pharmaceutical industry, but a few ones finally found valuable large scale applications in the food industry. Keys for the scale-up of well-known extraction and fractionation processes, together with examples of applications are discussed briefly. After a short reminder of the various SCF-based particle engineering processes described in the literature, the scale-up issues of these particle engineering processes for industrial applications are detailed. The discussed features then focus on pharmaceutical industry peculiar requirements, such as compliance with current Good Manufacturing Practices (cGMP). Finally, examples of recent applications, together with cost estimations, are given.

INTRODUCTION

Among scientific fields investigated over the last 50 years, the use of supercritical (SC) fluids (SCF) was probably seen as one of the most promising and universally applicable techniques for a variety of applications: solvent free extraction and fractionation, particle design and engineering, chromatography, reactions, sterilization… These perspectives raised considerable academic and industrial efforts for bringing the supercritical fluid technology to maturity in each investigated field. By extension, the SCF acronym will herein be used for fluids operated either in supercritical conditions or in near-critical conditions, the fluid being in compressed liquid or dense gas state.

The use of supercritical fluids at industrial scale started in the early 1970s as so-called extraction processes for solid feeds and fractionation processes for liquid feeds mainly in the food industry. To date, most SCF industrial units in the world are still using one of these processes mostly for the food and flavor industry but with continuously growing applications in the nutraceutical and pharmaceutical fields. Consequently, scale-up rules for extraction and fractionation processes are now well established for a wide number of products and will be only briefly discussed here.

Claimed in the 1990s as a promising universal toolbox for particle design and engineering for pharmaceutical applications, industrial use of supercritical fluids for particle formation is still exclusively applied for food ingredients and, to our knowledge, there are no examples of approved and marketed products in the pharmaceutical field. Nevertheless, as underlined in a recent review of high-pressure micronization processes for particle formation [1], it can be reasonably considered that the SCF particle engineering technology is now mature for some food applications and that so formulated pharmaceutical products will consequently reach the market within the next decade. The following review will thus mainly focus on scale-up issues for particle engineering processes in the pharmaceutical field with particular attention to cGMP requirements and their consequences in terms of design and implementation of full-scale units.

SCALE-UP KEYS

Supercritical Fluids Used At Industrial Scale

Carbon dioxide is the most attractive and used supercritical fluid at industrial scale. It is a low cost fluid, widely abundant in pure form, non flammable, not toxic (although it requires specific safety precautions [2]), and environment-friendly. Carbon dioxide critical point (31°C – 74 bar) allows operations at moderate temperature and accessible pressures (the maximal operating pressure is usually set at 300 bar for the most current full scale units and up to 1000 bar for the most recent ones). Some industrial plants use light hydrocarbons, especially propane [3] which is not toxic but flammable. Other types of fluids are or were also investigated for specific applications such as hydrofluorocarbons (HFCs), and especially 1,1,1,2-tetrafluoroethane (R134a), although they present high global warming power (1,430 for R134a versus 1 for CO_2) [4] and are more expensive than CO_2. Recent investigations use dimethylether in liquefied gas state, with ability to dissolve a wider range of compounds than usual SCFs [5].

Safety Issues

Specific attention is required when handling supercritical fluids and liquefied gases since significant hazards are resulting from their use [2]. In particular, safety must be considered as the main priority at each step of equipment design, building, installation, operation and maintenance. In addition, a detailed analysis of potential hazards should be conducted for any case. It must be also understood that on a versatile plant such as commonly used for extraction or fractionation but also for almost all particle engineering units, each new product treated in the unit must be considered as a new case with product specific safety aspects to be dealt with.

The main hazards to be considered are the following:

- Mechanical hazards,

- Thermodynamic hazards,

- Chemical hazards,

- Biological hazards,

When rigorously following design standards and applying tests and required inspections for high-pressure units by the local authorities, mechanical hazards can be mastered. Particularly, metal fatigue or brittle fracture risks must be taken into account especially for large scale units where the vessels are commonly built in carbon steel covered by an internal stainless steel cladding. Metal fatigue must be considered when designing the unit. Brittle fracture may arise either from corrosion due to the presence of water with CO_2 in the vessel (which cannot be avoided when handling natural products) or from steel phase induced by temperatures below -20°C when the vessels are depressurized too quickly. Frequent and strict inspections of the vessels are therefore mandatory and vessels life duration must be defined in terms of pressurization/depressurization cycles (typically 20,000).

Regarding thermodynamic hazards, ice or dry ice formation must be considered. For all the currently used supercritical fluids and of particular relevance with carbon dioxide, drastic temperature decreases are to be expected upon depressurization. A strong temperature drop may lead to solidification of water or products and to dry ice formation, resulting in potentially dangerous plugging of filters, tubing, vent lines... Consequently, as a general rule, specific areas where such plugging may occur must be clearly identified during the design, built carefully and frequently inspected/cleaned. BLEVE (Boiling Liquid Expanding Vapor Explosion) must also be considered [6]. The sudden rupture of the vessel itself may induce brutal release of the liquefied gas or supercritical fluid to the atmosphere and subsequent BLEVE. Damages caused by this phenomenon will increase when flammable gases are used. Frequently inspected sealing devices and safety devices such as fire detectors and safety valves allow to reduce significantly opportunities for BLEVE formation.

Chemical hazards in the supercritical technology are to be considered when flammable supercritical fluids, co-solvents or products are involved. Even if carbon dioxide is largely used in the food industry for extraction and fractionation, it is often used in combination with a flammable co-solvent, ethanol being the most common one. Consequently, equipment and buildings must generally be designed at least for avoiding co-solvent vapor accumulation. When using flammable supercritical fluids, explosion proof plants have to be designed and drastic safety procedures must be implemented.

Supercritical fluids may induce biological hazards by themselves. Despite its low toxicity and as for all inert gases, carbon dioxide can cause asphyxia. Particular care must be taken in the design of the buildings in order to avoid the accumulation of gaseous carbon dioxide, heavier than air, especially in underground passages and cellars. Installation of gas detectors in appropriate areas is mandatory.

In addition, there is always a high level of risk associated with handling of biologically active products (fluid, co-solvent, raw material or extract from the raw material) when operating supercritical fluid units. At any time, fluid leakage may lead to easily inhaled aerosol. As a general rule when handling highly active or toxic products, it is recommended to isolate the plant in a well-vented closed environment possibly with remote control or at least with permanent respiratory protection of the operators and to implement an efficient treatment of the vented gases exiting the unit. Treatment of the vented gases needs to be designed either for normal venting operations but also for emergency releases with appropriate containment of the contaminated vented gases, scrubbing and/or filtration prior to fluid recycle or release to the atmosphere. The presence of high concentration of biologically active products is commonly dealt with in the pharmaceutical field, but it may also be an unexpected issue when handling natural products containing low levels of potent compounds concentrated throughout the supercritical process.

The operational safety of supercritical fluid processing plant is generally ensured through appropriate design especially redundancy of the safety elements, taking into account any identified potential hazard (fire, electrical power, utilities or ancillaries failure...). As for most of the processes, incidents or accidents arise from risk underestimation or misunderstanding by the operators and appropriate training is a major key in the safe operation of units. Particularly, peculiar issues may be underestimated by the operators especially on versatile units such as R&D multipurpose equipment or multi-product commercial scale processing unit. For example, plugging of piping or extraction baskets may happen with particular products prone to melt or plasticize under SCF processing conditions (polymers, highly viscous extracts, waxes...). Such products may foam, expand or solidify upon depressurization with consecutive risks of damage to the unit itself and/or serious injuries to the operators [7].

Scale-Up of Scf Processes: Fluid Management Issues

As a general recommendation for SCF processing units and of particular relevance for large scale SCF plants, fluid management requires particular attention, including fluid supply, storage and delivery, fluid recycling and/or disposal [8].

For example, high purity carbon dioxide ($\geq$ 99.5%) can be easily supplied in large amounts and generally fulfils the requirements for SFE and SFF applications. Usual impurities in carbon dioxide (moisture, nitrogen, oxygen, methane, hydrocarbons) are not of particular concern for such applications. However, when high added value products at very low concentrations in the raw material are to be recovered or for nutraceutical/pharmaceutical applications, non volatile organic pollutants may become an issue since they may contaminate the final product at significant levels. More stringent carbon dioxide specifications and peculiar controls are then required.

On-site storage of the fluid in liquid state may also be a source of contamination if not properly designed, cleaned and operated. For carbon dioxide, stainless steel instead of carbon steel storage tanks are recommended, otherwise rust formation and subsequent product contamination may occur even at low moisture contents.

Energy and fluid requirements for the fluid cycle depend on one side of the raw material and the chosen operating conditions (mainly pressure and temperature) and on the other side on the mode of carrying out the fluid cycle. For obvious economical and ecological reasons, the fluid is preferentially recycled on large scale extraction and fractionation units. Consequently, separation of solute(s) from the fluid must be optimized both in terms of energy consumption and in terms of fluid purity in the recycling loop in order to avoid product deposition and resulting heat exchange efficiency reduction or even plugging.

Fluid disposal is generally operated by venting to the atmosphere which was already discussed above as a safety issue. For peculiar applications either with highly toxic compounds or alternative SCF such as R134a, potentially contaminated fluid recovery at the plant exit, storage and further destruction can be required.

EXTRACTION-FRACTIONATION

As already mentioned, the use of supercritical fluids in extraction (SFE) and fractionation (SFF) processes has been studied and implemented at large scale for almost 40 years. General chemical engineering rules for the design of extraction and fractionation industrial scale units together with examples of applications are described in details throughout literature [9,10]. Thermodynamic modeling, simulation and optimization of SFE and SFF processes has also been reviewed recently [11].

Design of SFE Full Scale Plants

Supercritical fluid extraction (SFE) processes (Fig. **1**) can be rather simply scaled-up from lab-scale or pilot-scale [12]. Following the determination of the optimal extraction conditions (pressure, temperature, solvent ratios and composition) through an appropriate design of experiments, the governing mechanism for the extraction process can be identified. Depending of the type of raw materials from which extraction is carried out, the process may be solubility driven, diffusion driven or both solubility and diffusion driven. For example, lipids are usually easy to extract from the raw material matrix leading to a predominantly solubility driven extraction process. On the contrary, solvent stripping or pesticide removal from raw materials is often diffusion limited. In most cases where the extraction process is both solubility and diffusion driven, scale-up may be achieved simply by keeping constant both the fresh raw material to SCF mass ratio and the SCF flow rate to raw material mass ratio (i.e. the SCF residence time in the vessel). More sophisticated numerical simulations based upon knowledge of the transport mechanism of the extract from the raw material to the SCF allow improved design of the industrial plant.

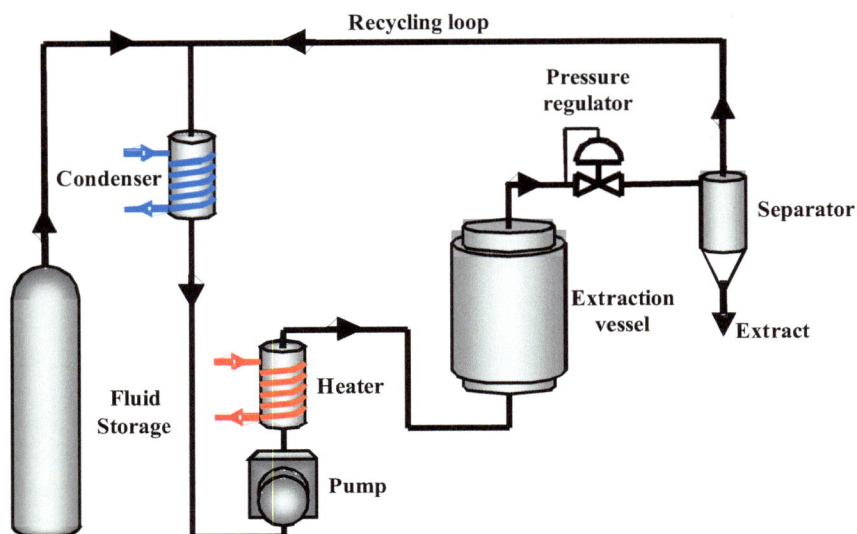

Figure 1: Schematic representation of a basic SFE unit.

Full scale extraction units are usually using batch processing composed of at least two extractors. However, the use of at least three extractors is to be preferred since continuous processing through simulated moving solid configurations can then be implemented. One of the extractor is under loading/discharge operation while the remaining ones are connected in series so that the contact between the SCF and the raw material is achieved with increased extraction efficiency.

Solid raw material preparation prior to loading of the extraction vessel requires particular care when operating large scale units. Most raw materials processed at industrial scale are natural products with a high degree of variability (shape, size, moisture, etc) for the same material depending on the source, the storage conditions… Without care, such variability may induce drastic changes in the extraction process efficiency between batches. For coarse dry products, preliminary grinding is usually recommended. Grinding must usually be completed by fine particles removal e.g. by sieving in order to avoid the occurrence of plugging of the extraction basket filters. Great care must also be taken when handling highly compressible and/or semi-solid raw materials since the weight of the material itself in the extraction basket may lead to caking issues with risks of reduced contact efficiency between the solvent and the material due to channeling or, in the worst case, plugging of the extraction basket filter. When semi-solid products are to be treated, their preliminary mixture with an inert material (cellulose for example) may help to resolve this issue.

Design of SFF Full Scale Plants

Supercritical fluid fractionation (SFF) industrial units (Fig. **2**) are usually operated continuously in a counter current column but may also be achieved in mixer-settler units for high SCF to feed flow rates or when density difference between the SCF and the liquid raw material is low, limiting the flow in a gravity driven column [3]. For the design of an industrial counter-current column, scale-up is complicated by the fact that column diameter increase may lead to increased axial mixing with dramatic effects on fractionation efficiency in terms of height equivalent to a theoretical plate.

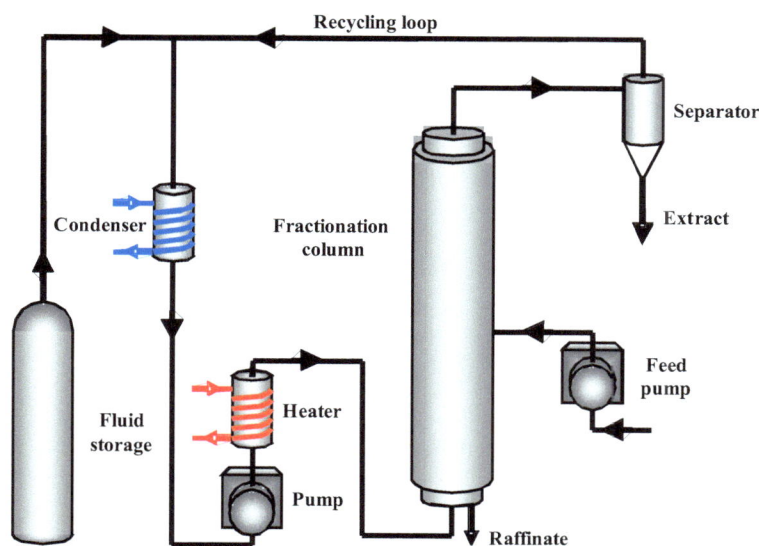

Figure 2: Schematic representation of a basic SFF unit.

Similarly to liquid-liquid extraction scale-up, the following experimental approach is recommended [8] before designing a SFF industrial unit. The liquid and SCF hold up curves are first determined at pilot-scale in the chosen experimental conditions (pressure, temperature and packing type) so that flow rates leading to flooding are identified. Flooding may also be induced by modification of the hydrodynamic pattern inside the column due to foaming, especially with natural products or fermentation derived products. Once the above mentioned curves are determined, the column diameter can be estimated, avoiding the zones where flooding may occur. Column length can then be evaluated taking into account the higher axial mixing phenomenon induced by column diameter increase. Particular care must also be paid to the design of the liquid and SCF distributors, knowing that channeling may be reduced by fractionating the packing in several beds separated by redistribution plates. As mentioned for SFE, raw material preparation may be of critical importance when operating with natural products in order to reduce variation between batches.

SFE and SFF Applications and Perspectives

Recent reviews of applications of SFE and SFF processes are of particular interest. Early, present and possible applications of counter-current separation [3] with supercritical fluids are detailed together with more peculiar applications to specialty lipids with near critical fluids [5] or supercritical processing of fats and oils [13]. The compilation of all possible and actual applications is outside the objective of the present review. Nevertheless, major identified fields of applications of fractionation can be cited from the above mentioned reviews: edible oil (from fish, seeds and nuts) components and derivatives, citrus oil and components, essential oils, flavors.

As a general rule, it can be stated that most SFF and SFE full scale plants are multi-product processing units for food and flavor industries. Except the pioneering full scale units such as the ones for caffeine removal from coffee beans and tea leaves and for hops extraction, only a few dedicated industrial plants have been erected for example for the de-oiling of lecithin with propane and for recovery of caffeine from water in a decaffeination cycle [3]. Another recent example in connection with the food industry is a unit with a capacity of 2,500 tons per year cork treatment for the removal of trichloroanisole, primarily responsible for cork taste in wine [14]. While environmental considerations, such as alternative to hexane use in some edible oils extraction, are one of the main driving forces for a wider use of SCF technology, the required handling of large volumes of oilseeds is still a major challenge when using SCF technology [13].

About 100 SFE full scale units with a total extraction volume above 500 liters were built in the world to date [15] with equal repartition of about 45 of these units in Europe and Asia and almost 15 units in America. Such plants are generally dedicated to large volume extraction from rather low value raw materials leading to significantly higher value products.

The main perspectives for SFE and SFF are presently oriented towards products with much higher added value than the ones upon which the SCF technology was developed at full scale in the past 30 years. More precisely, most recent potential full scale applications are targeting products for functionalized foods, nutraceuticals or even pharmaceuticals. For example, extraction and fractionation of specialty lipids such as high-value seed oils containing polyunsaturated fatty acids already found some commercial success and efforts are currently focusing on concentration of polyunsaturated fatty acids or their direct extraction from micro-organisms [5].

Finally, there is a general and recent agreement to state that SFE and SFF future applications will no longer be operated as single-step operations but as integrated unit operations [13,16] either in combination with usual techniques such as membrane separation or with processes also involving SCF technology such as high-pressure reactors or particle formation units.

PARTICLE ENGINEERING

Drivers of SCF Particle Engineering in the Food and Pharmaceutical Industry

SCF-based processes actually offer new opportunities to meet the challenge of producing high purity, chemically and physically stable micro- or nano-particles with low solvent residues, controlled morphology and tailored properties [17-19]. As recently reviewed [1], similar drivers exist for the development of SCF particle design processes for food applications. Food products with enhanced properties or with superior quality to the state of the art have already been produced in large SCF plants.

The major aim of processing pharmaceuticals with SCF processes is to obtain particulate dry materials with a desired particle size distribution, morphology, physical form and crystallinity. Preferably, this goal is achieved through a one-step process enabling to avoid a laborious downstream processing (drying, reduction of residual solvent content...). Indeed, most of the final dosage forms require drug substances in a particulate form with specific size distribution, physico-chemical properties and solid state morphology.

It is now established that a major challenge of the pharmaceutical industry is to deal with poorly soluble drugs which are frequently associated with a poor and variable bioavailability [20]. Basically, the absorption of a drug administered by the oral route is related to its apparent solubility in the intestinal fluid and its ability to cross the intestinal barrier [21]. Therefore, for poorly soluble drugs, one of the key issues to enhance absorption, and hence bioavailability, is to increase the dissolution rate and/or the solubility in the gastrointestinal fluids. Particle size which controls surface area is one of the parameters which govern dissolution rate in the gastrointestinal fluids. Size reduction of active pharmaceutical ingredients (APIs) so as to engineer the drug itself in micro- or nano-particulate form has thus emerged as a major strategy for the pharmaceutical industry. The solid state morphology (i.e. polymorphism and crystallinity) of drug substances has also an impact on dissolution rate and apparent solubility of drugs [22]. One further interest of micronization, or nanosizing, of a drug is that it makes it often possible to consider a more appropriate and convenient administration route than the usual one. For instance, pharmaceutical powders less than 5 μm in size can be used in aerosols for respiratory delivery of drugs. Inhaled drugs need to be micronized by suitable techniques [23], producing particles within the target range of 1-5 μm and with optimal surface properties and solid state morphology.

The formation of drug-loaded composite particles with tailored size, morphology and composition is also an increasing challenge for therapeutic applications. The processing of composites is of major interest to develop innovative therapeutic systems such as oral solid dispersions [24] with enhanced rate of dissolution, inclusion complexes employing cyclodextrins [25], polymer particles [26] as injectable sustained-release formulations of fragile biomolecules In solid dispersions, the drug is typically dispersed (molecularly or not) in a hydrophilic polymer matrix, and released in form of colloidal particles in the gastrointestinal tract. With peculiar excipients, solid dispersions are also used to control and slow the drug release for oral formulations. Composite particles are also particularly suitable to provide injectable sustained-release delivery systems. Basically, drug-containing polymer or lipid particles with a size typically lower than 100 µm can be injected subcutaneously to obtain sustained-release depots [27]. Drug-containing polymer nanoparticles, whose size is lower than 1 µm, can be administered intravenously to increase the systemic circulating time of the drug, reduce its toxicity and target solid tumors according to the enhanced permeability and retention (EPR) effect in tumor vasculature [28,29].

However, finely powdered pharmaceuticals and composite particles are often difficult to produce in a reliable way by currently available drying or micronization techniques, thus hindering the development of these promising formulations. These techniques, such as spray-drying [30], operate at temperatures that can thermally induce chemical degradation of thermolabile drugs or denaturation of heat-sensitive compounds, such as proteins. In the same way, milling, which is one of the currently used techniques for comminuting drug particles, suffers from disadvantages such as lack of control over the size, shape and surface properties of the milled particles, and a high energy input that can possibly affect the stability, polymorphism and degree of crystallinity of the drug [31].

As regards the manufacturing of drug nanoparticles, various innovative techniques have been successfully applied [32]: aerosol flow reactor method, microemulsion template technology, media milling (e.g. Nanocrystal® technology), high-pressure homogenization (e.g. DissoCubes®), and continuous precipitation techniques. Some of these innovative techniques rely on the use of organic solvents and/or stringent operating conditions, limiting their application to a narrow range of drug substance. Milder nanosizing processes such as media milling and high-pressure homogenization can be used for a wide range of APIs (thermolabile, poorly soluble in both aqueous or organic media), but end up with nanoparticle suspensions, hence leading to a complex downstream processing when a dry solid dosage form is required.

It is also worthwhile noticing that current methods for preparation of composite drug micro- or nano-particles are laborious and often poorly reproducible. These methods are mainly solvent-based techniques, such as co-precipitation or cosolvent evaporation, emulsion-solvent extraction, phase separation, spray-drying. Other methods are based on hot-melt procedures, such as hot-melt extrusion or hot-melt emulsification. Manufacturing of cyclodextrin inclusion complexes also relies on solvent-based and stringent processes: kneading, co-evaporation, co-milling. These techniques exhibit the same drawbacks as those quoted above for pure pharmaceutical compounds, related to potential degradation of fragile drugs and toxicity of residual solvents.

Available SCF Particle Engineering Processes for Food and Pharmaceutical Applications

Several SCF processes have been reported in the literature for the generation of tailored particles [19]:

- Rapid Expansion from Supercritical Solutions (RESS) [33], in which particles are precipitated from a SC solution, due to high supersaturation ratios caused by rapid expansion.

- Gas Anti-Solvent (GAS) [34] and Supercritical Anti-Solvent (SAS), in which The SCF (usually CO_2) is used as an anti-solvent which causes precipitation of the material initially dissolved in an organic solvent. This process has many related modifications (Aerosol Solvent Extraction System: ASES process, Solution Enhanced Dispersion by SCF: SEDS process, etc) [19,35].

- Generation of Particles from Gas-Saturated Solutions (PGSS) [36] and related processes, in which SC CO_2 is used as a swelling, viscosity-reducing and plasticizing agent dissolved in the material. The so-formed gas-saturated solution is further expanded through a nozzle to cause particle precipitation. A closely related process, the so-called Concentrated Powder Form (CPF) [37] allows generating free flowing powders loaded with a high content of liquid by contacting a liquid with a pressurized gas, expanding the mixture in a nozzle then contacting the finely dispersed spray with a solid carrier material.

Other currently investigated processes are also very promising for the manufacturing of food or pharmaceutical formulations, such as the controlled impregnations of polymer with drugs dissolved in supercritical fluids [38] or deposition of drugs onto porous preformed carriers [39], Supercritical Fluid Extraction of Emulsions (SFEE) leading to the recovery of drug particles or drug-loaded composite particles dispersed in a liquid phase [40], depressurization of an expanded liquid organic solution (DELOS) crystallization technique [41], or coating of preformed particles obtained by a controlled phase separation of a coating agent dissolved in the SCF [42]. Some promising processes, consisting in a combination between established formulation processes and supercritical techniques have been recently developed, such as the hot-melt extrusion of polymers using pressurized CO_2 as a plasticizer and foaming agent [43]. Despite the promising results reported with these processes, we will herein focus on the features, scale-up issues and commercial applications of the three main SCF particle design techniques, namely RESS, SC anti-solvent processes, PGSS and its closely related processes.

RESS

Production of particles by RESS relies on the fact that the solvent strength of a SCF can be dramatically reduced by altering its pressure. The expansion of a SC solution to ambient pressure leads to high supersaturation, nucleation and consequently to the formation of fine particles [19,25,44].

RESS allows the production of solvent-free particles within a single-step operation and can be implemented in a simple way. As presented in Fig. 3, the RESS process consists in dissolving the material to be powdered in a SCF, heating the SC solution to the desired pre-expansion temperature then expanding the SC solution through a nozzle into a low pressure chamber.

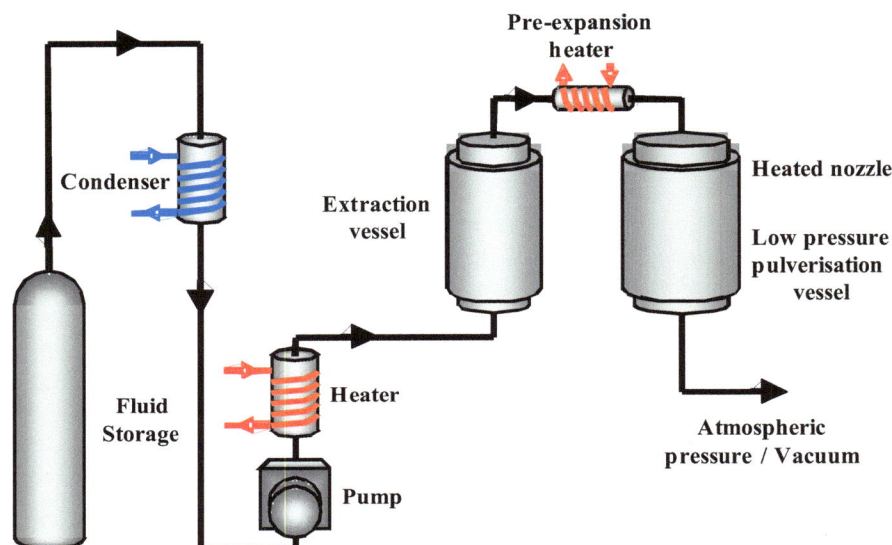

Figure 3: Schematic representation of a RESS unit.

Apart from the utilities dedicated to the supply and transfer of the pressurized SCF, a RESS unit is composed of high-pressure vessels used to dissolve the material to be powdered into the SCF, possibly a pre-expansion heater and a low pressure vessel where the supercritical solution is expanded through a heated nozzle typically at near-ambient pressure. The supercritical solution must be heated before expansion so as to prevent condensation of the fluid upon expansion, the pre-expansion temperature being set by heating the nozzle and frequently with an additional preheating device. For thermally labile materials, such as active pharmaceutical ingredients, thermal stability issues may occur due to the rather high required pre-expansion temperatures (at least 100°C with CO_2 for usual extraction pressures above 200 bar).

Various solid shapes and morphologies are obtained using the RESS process, from fine powders to needles, as illustrated by the micronisation of lovastatin, an anti-cholesterol drug, by RESS with CO_2 (Fig. **4**). Starting from large and irregular particles, either porous agglomerates of nano-particles, or micro-particles in form of spheres or of rod crystals were obtained. Moreover, provided that both the drug and the excipients are soluble in the supercritical fluid, the RESS process can be applied to the engineering of drug-loaded composite particles. Only few examples of co-precipitation by RESS were reported [45-47]. These results clearly showed that the formation of composite microparticles with a low molecular weight pharmaceutical or nutraceutical compound incorporated within a bioresorbable polymer matrix can be achieved using the RESS process with CO_2, but for a restricted range of drug/carrier systems, due to the low solubility of most of APIs and excipients in supercritical CO_2, narrowing the field of potential therapeutic applications.

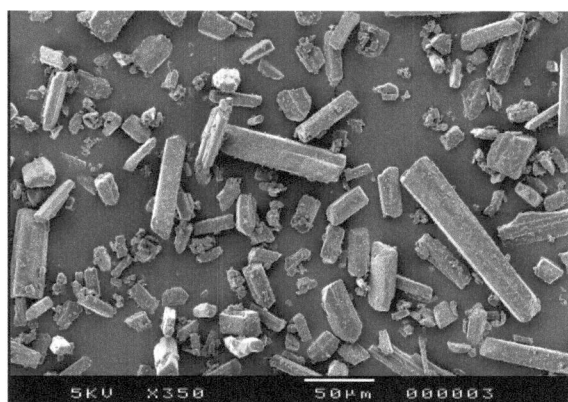

a) Raw Lovastatin

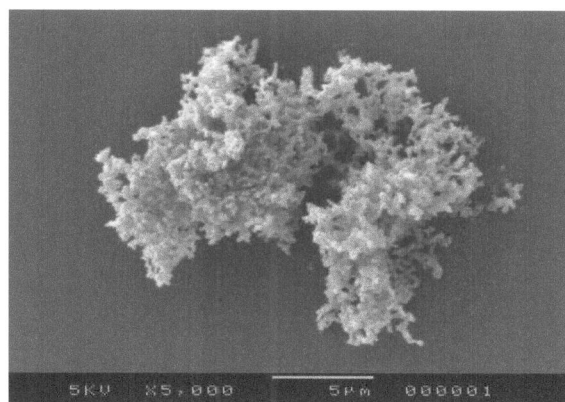

b) Lovastatin nano-particles

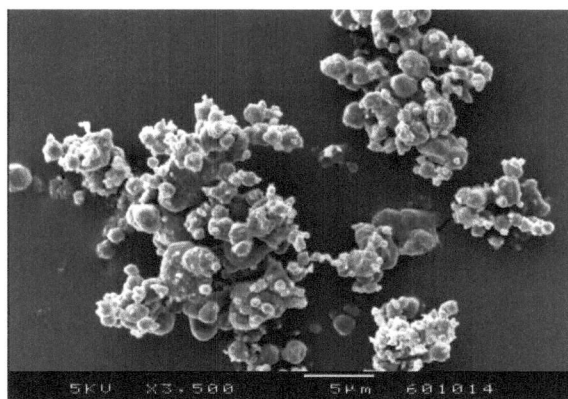

c) Micronised lovastatin

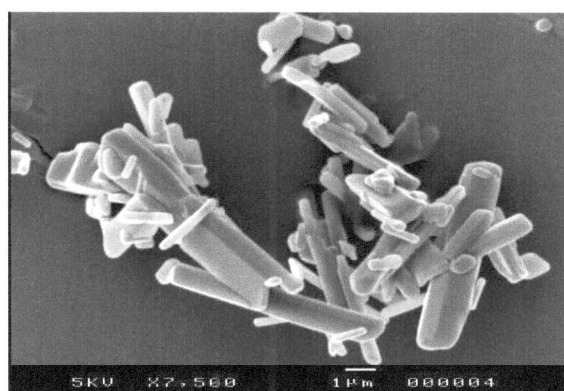

d) Micronised lovastatin

Figure 4: Micronization of lovastatin by RESS (*Courtesy of Separex*)

As pointed out in a recent review of experimental research on the RESS process, the relationship between the process conditions and the particle properties is still unclear [44]. Apart from the SCF nature and the solute to be precipitated, the main operating parameters which influence the particulate product morphology are the extraction and pre-expansion temperature and pressure which define the thermodynamic pathway of the RESS process and the nozzle geometry and diameter. Depending on the nature of solutes and operating conditions, the RESS process can produce very small and nearly monodisperse nanoparticles [48,49]. Nevertheless, due to particle aggregation during free jet expansion and post-expansion residence time, microparticulate fractions are often generated. The aggregation rate of the particles can be minimized by expanding the SC solution into an aqueous solution containing a surfactant which impedes the particle growth and agglomeration. Using such a modified process known as RESAS [50] and polysorbitan ester as surfactant, aqueous dispersions of cyclosporine nanoparticles whose size ranged ~ 400 – 700 nm, were produced. Nevertheless, this modified RESS process leads to the recovery of a nanoparticle dispersion in a liquid continuous phase with similar drawbacks to the above mentioned more conventional processes as regards the downstream processing to produce a solid dosage form. In addition, dry nano-/micro-particles often exhibit unfavorable physical properties leading to difficult handling and downstream processing to produce the final dosage form (tablets, capsules). In order to overcome these issues, an innovative approach has been developed: the micronized particles generated by the RESS process are collected on a water-soluble excipient bed [51], as illustrated in Fig. **5** for RESS-micronized lovastatin trapped onto lactose granules. The dry formulation can be handled without dust emission as a free-flowing powder and was found to be readily processable so as to produce final solid dosage form such as tablets. RESS could find valuable applications at the commercial scale only when the product solubility in the supercritical fluid is not too small, typically $\geq 10^{-4}$ kg/kg, drastically limiting its application when CO_2 is used as solvent. Hence it is considered that the RESS process is suitable for high value materials, excluding many food ingredients. Today the most promising applications of RESS processing are thus related to the processing of active pharmaceutical ingredients: nanosized drugs for parenteral administration, microparticles for inhalation, nano- or micro-particlesfor oral administration of poorly soluble drugs. However, recent works demonstrated that a much wider range of molecules could be processed by RESS when using fluids such as dimethylether [5,52]

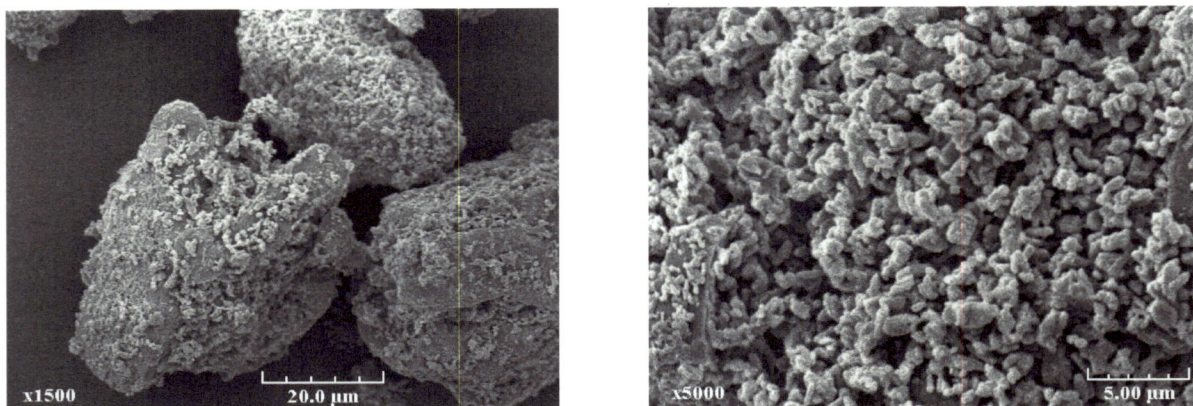

Figure 5: RESS-micronized Lovastatin microparticles trapped on lactose particles (*Courtesy of Separex*)

SC Anti-Solvent Processes

Liquid anti-solvent processes are widely used to precipitate, purify or micronize various substrates. Starting from an organic solution, the addition of a miscible anti-solvent induces supersaturation and precipitation of the solute. Attributes of a good anti-solvent include high diffusivity, low viscosity, and high solubility within the solvent, which are all consistent with the properties of SC CO_2. One further advantage of SC anti-solvents is that they are easily removed by a simple pressure decrease, while the removal of liquid anti-solvent is difficult and requires a complex and costly downstream elimination procedure. SCF anti-solvent processes have thus been extensively studied as alternatives to liquid anti-solvent processes. At the laboratory scale, SC anti-solvent processes allowed the formation of particles with controlled size and morphology from a wide range of compounds, including water-soluble compounds such as therapeutic proteins [53,54].

Two modes of operations may be implemented for SC anti-solvent processes: static batch processes and semi-continuous spray-based processes.

The static gas anti-solvent process (GAS) involves the injection of CO_2 into a high-pressure vessel loaded with a liquid solution (Fig. **6**). The gradual addition of CO_2 expands the liquid solution and induces supersaturation and precipitation of the solute initially dissolved in the organic solution. Once the solute has been precipitated, the suspension of particles must be drained with a flow of supercritical fluid to eliminate the liquid organic solvent before depressurization and collection of particles. At the laboratory scale, various pharmaceuticals were crystallized by GAS [19].

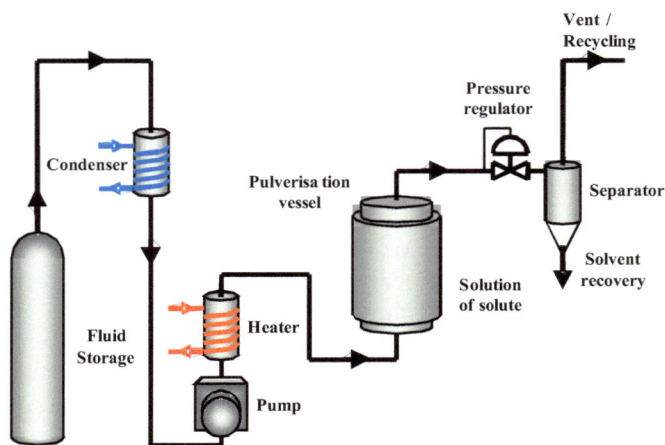

Figure 6: Schematic representation of a GAS unit (static batch process)

The SC anti-solvent processes are also operated in a semi-continuous way; the liquid solution is sprayed through a nozzle into, or with, compressed CO_2 in a high pressure vessel (Fig. 7). SC CO_2 is also fed in the high pressure vessel via a high pressure pump. After production of particles, SC CO_2 must flow through the vessel to remove residual solvents from the microparticles. These spray processes have been called PCA (Precipitation with Compressed Anti-solvent) [55], SAS (Supercritical Anti-solvent), ASES (Aerosol Solvent Extraction System) [56], or SEDS (Supercritical Enhanced Dispersion by Supercritical fluid

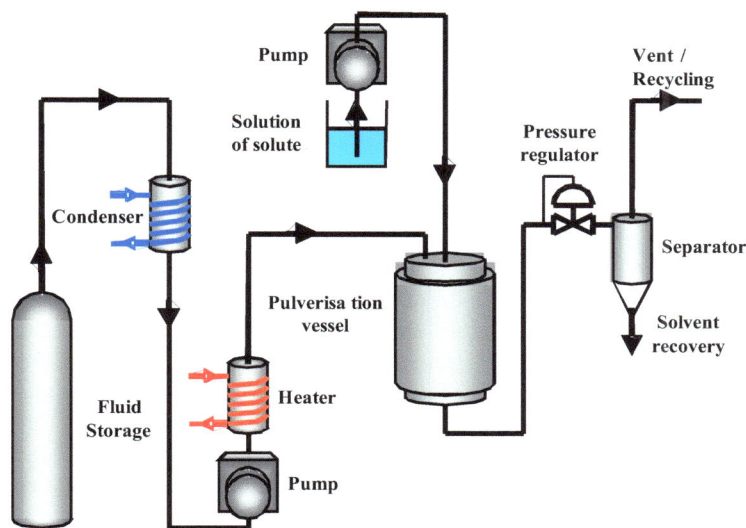

Figure 7: Schematic representation of a SAS/PCA/ASES/SEDS unit (semi-continuous spray-based process) [57].

Various parameters have an influence on the morphology and size of particles produced by SC anti-solvent processes. More particularly, influencing parameters are the nozzle design, the flow rates of SCF and liquid solutions, the pressure and the temperature, the solution concentration, the spraying velocity, the residence time of particles in the high pressure vessel [58-61]. A comprehensive understanding of anti-solvent precipitation should include contributions from thermodynamics, hydrodynamics, mass transfer and precipitation kinetics, with many unresolved problems concerning the dispersion or mixing in such environment and also the process of local supersaturation, nucleation and surface integration.

A variety of precipitate morphologies have been found to result from the spray-based SC anti-solvent processes (Fig. 8) such as microspheres, fibers, hollow microspheres and interconnected networks. Numerous examples of particle design showed that the particle morphology can be tuned, including the generation of a specific crystal patterns in case of polymorphism [62-64].

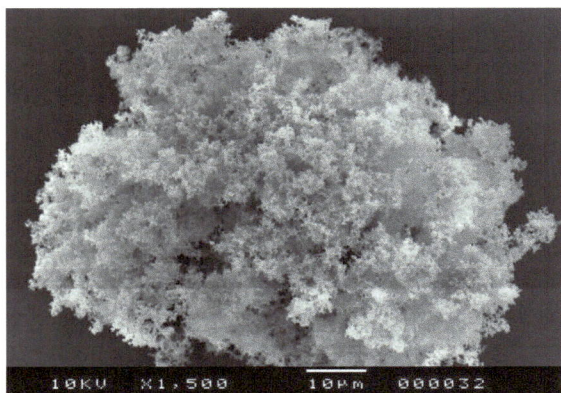

a) Atorvastatin nano-particles   b) Atorvastatin micro-particles

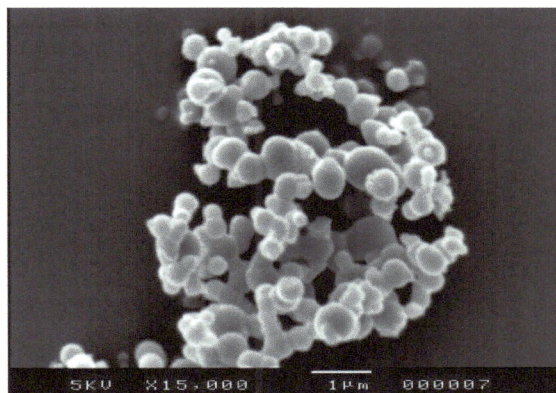

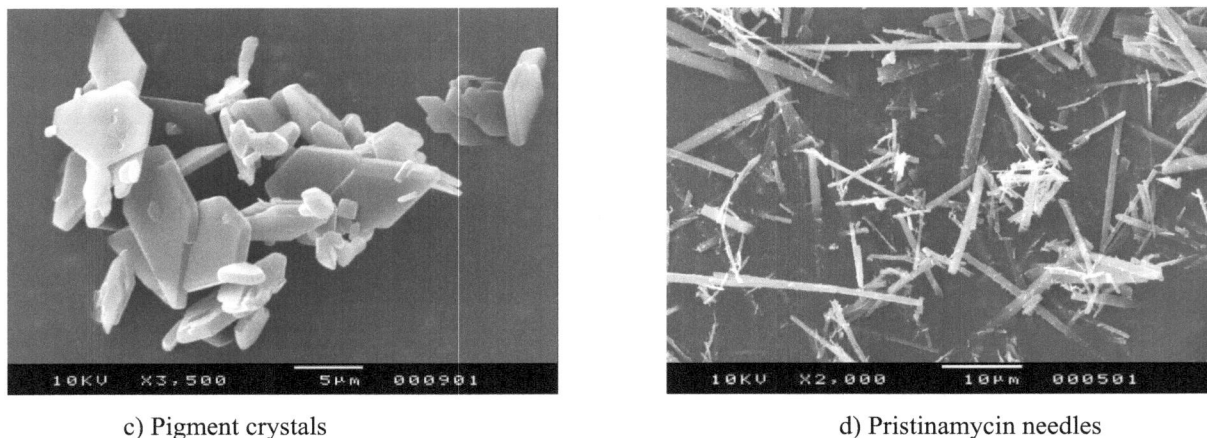

c) Pigment crystals

d) Pristinamycin needles

Figure 8: Micronization by anti-solvent (*Courtesy of Separex*)

SC anti-solvent processes are also suitable for the preparation of drug-loaded composite particles. Indeed, starting from liquid solutions of drugs and carriers, these processes make feasible the co-precipitation of both the active drug and the carrier from one or two liquid solutions sprayed in the anti-solvent. Co-precipitation of poorly soluble drugs and solubilizing excipients according to the SC antisolvent processes has been reported as a promising way to produce solid dispersions exhibiting an improved dissolution rate [65-67]. Regarding the manufacturing of drug-loaded polymer particles for controlled-release formulations, the Tg depression and polymer softening in presence of CO_2 of polymers used for controlled-release application (e.g. poly(lactic acid-co-glycolic acid) (PLGA) copolymers) was reported as a major concern. These polymers often soften in

the precipitation vessel and lead to agglomeration, adhesion to the precipitation vessel walls or formation of films. Hence, the encapsulation of drugs with a large range of bioerodible polymer composition and molecular weight, together with a high drug loading efficiency still remains a challenge using SC antisolvent processes.

SC anti-solvent processes have also been successfully implemented for the production of inclusion complexes of drugs and cyclodextrins (CD's). A solution of the active drug and a CD derivative in an organic solvent, was atomized into a stream of SCF solvent leading to controlled-size particles with a high degree of complexation of the drug resulting in a drastic increase of apparent solubility of the drug in water [51,68-70]. As regards the production of drug/cyclodextrins inclusion complexes, SCFs can be also used as vector for drug inclusion [71,71].

With regards to food applications, some SC anti-solvent related processes have been demonstrated to have industrial potential, as illustrated by the recent start-up of a production plant dedicated to the deoiling of soybean raw lecithin [1]. Raw lecithin, a liquid material containing about 60% phospholipids and 40% of oil where the oil acts as a solvent for phospholipids, is sprayed via a nozzle in a high-pressure vessel containing supercritical CO_2. This process is related to a pioneer process called high-pressure jet extraction [73] where the oily part of lecithin was extracted upon intimate mixing with supercritical CO_2, leading to the precipitation of the deoiled lecithin as a solid material. It has been reported that an industrial plant makes it possible to produce about 120 kg/h of deoiled lecithin powder which is withdrawn from the high-pressure vessel via a special lock device [74].

PGSS

Generation of Particles from gas-saturated solutions (PGSS) [36] involves the decompression of a solute-rich liquid phase in which the SCF is dissolved. The solubility of near-critical or SC CO_2 in liquids or melts is usually high, even for substances poorly soluble in SC CO_2. In addition upon contact with SC CO_2, several solid solutes, such as polymers [75,76] or lipids [77,78] can be melted, softened, swollen or plasticized. For instance, the sorption of CO_2 into many amorphous or semi-crystalline polymers leads to a dramatic decrease in the glass transition temperature (Tg) and a subsequent swelling of the polymer [79]. In addition, the viscosity of CO_2 expanded melts has been reported to be reduced by several orders of magnitude [80].

The first step of the PGSS process (Fig. **9**) involves the mixing of a SCF, generally CO_2, with a melted or liquid-suspended material to form a so-called gas-saturated solution or suspension. The mixture is further expanded through a nozzle to form fine droplets. Due to the Joule-Thomson effect, a sharp temperature decrease is caused by fluid expansion leading to solidification of the droplets.

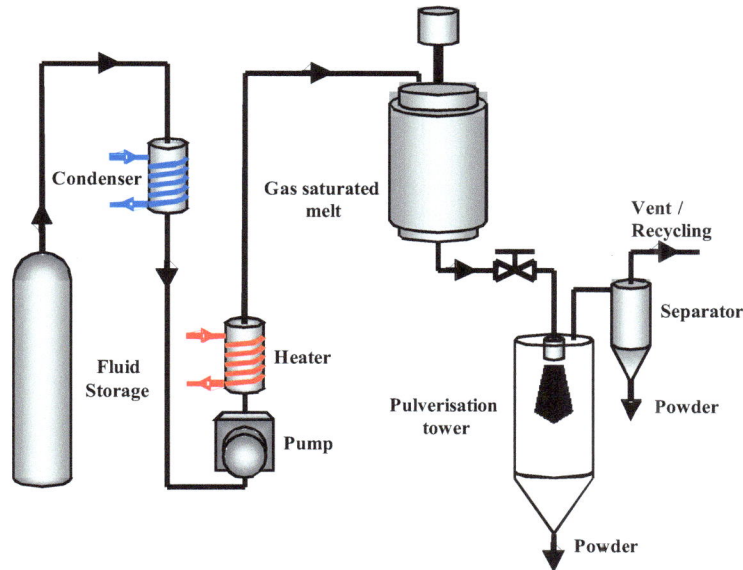

Figure 9: Schematic representation of a PGSS unit

For pharmaceutical applications, the PGSS process was mainly investigated with polymers and lipids, and scarcely applied to the production of pure drug particles, since PGSS processing of pure drugs involves operating at relatively high temperatures. Conversely, several food and food related products have been successfully powderized with the PGSS process: lecithin and phospholipids, glycerides, cocoa butter, fats, waxes, phytosterols.

Due to the swelling and plasticizing effect of supercritical CO_2 on high-molecular weight compounds such as polymers, PGSS, and related processes such as Fluid-Assisted

MicroEncapsulation (FAME), are particularly suitable for the production of composite particles such as solid dispersions of poorly soluble drugs into hydrophilic polymers so as to enhance their oral bioavailability. When applied to the production of drug-loaded polymer or lipid microspheres, the PGSS concept involves the expansion of a solution of the drug in the melted polymer, restricting its application to a few APIs which can be dissolved in the melted polymer. However, in variants of PGSS [81,82], the drug particles are dispersed in the liquefied carrier, allowing the processing of a wide range of drugs, provided that the drug is readily available as a fine powder.

Industrial Considerations for SCF Particle Design Processes Scale-Up

As reported hereinabove, the main pharmaceutical or food applications of SCF which have been developed at the industrial scale are related to extraction and fractionation processes. However, beside these well-known applications, strong and fast developments are under progress in the field of particle design. For the processing of pharmaceuticals, most of the promising SCF particle design techniques, and formulations obtained according to these processes, have been only reported at laboratory scale, or pilot scale for the manufacturing of clinical batches. Conversely, SCF particle design has been introduced industrially for food applications, as illustrated by the various applications of the PGSS or CPF processes.

Regarding pharmaceutical applications, a convincing evaluation of the biopharmaceutical performance of SCF-processed formulations, even at the earliest stages of development (proof of concept in animals, stability, tolerance), requires the ability to produce a sufficient amount of particles in a validated way, at least at the pilot scale. It is therefore not surprising that very few published works have assessed the biopharmaceutical performance of such formulations, slowing down the spreading of these promising processes in the pharmaceutical industry. The production of drug particles or drug-loaded particles by SCF processes has to fulfill the following three major requirements to envision a widespread use of these unique techniques:

(i). safety of operation: this remains a major concern as SCF processes are connected with the treatment of biologically active materials in a high-pressure environment;

(ii). as any industrial process, SCF processes have to be scaled up with acceptable production costs and a high reliability;

(iii).the production under cGMP standards, with important concerns about the cleanability of units and the purity of process fluids.

As already underlined when discussing general safety issues related to SCF processes scaling-up, the generation of bioactive particles with high-pressure processes gives rise to specific safety issues which have to be addressed to ensure the development of SC processes in the pharmaceutical industry [83]. The high-pressure processing conditions favor the formation of aerosols resulting from leaks or fast depressurization. This contamination hazard by aerosols is obviously of major concern for pharmaceutical potent products. It is thus mandatory that a high level of containment is used to reduce the risk of contamination of the working area and environment. Protection of the pharmaceutical product from any contamination is also a key-issue referring to GMP. These two constraints must be combined when designing the pressure map inside a clean room receiving a high-pressure equipment, and its access rooms (Fig. **10**). The main non-accidental hazard is related to particle release at the end of the run when the powder has to be recovered. This issue is addressed by a careful design of the equipment, particularly of the atomization vessel from where the atomized powder shall be extracted without external release. Moreover, the transfer of the particles to a safe container shall be operated inside a laminar-flow hood with complete filtration of the effluent air.

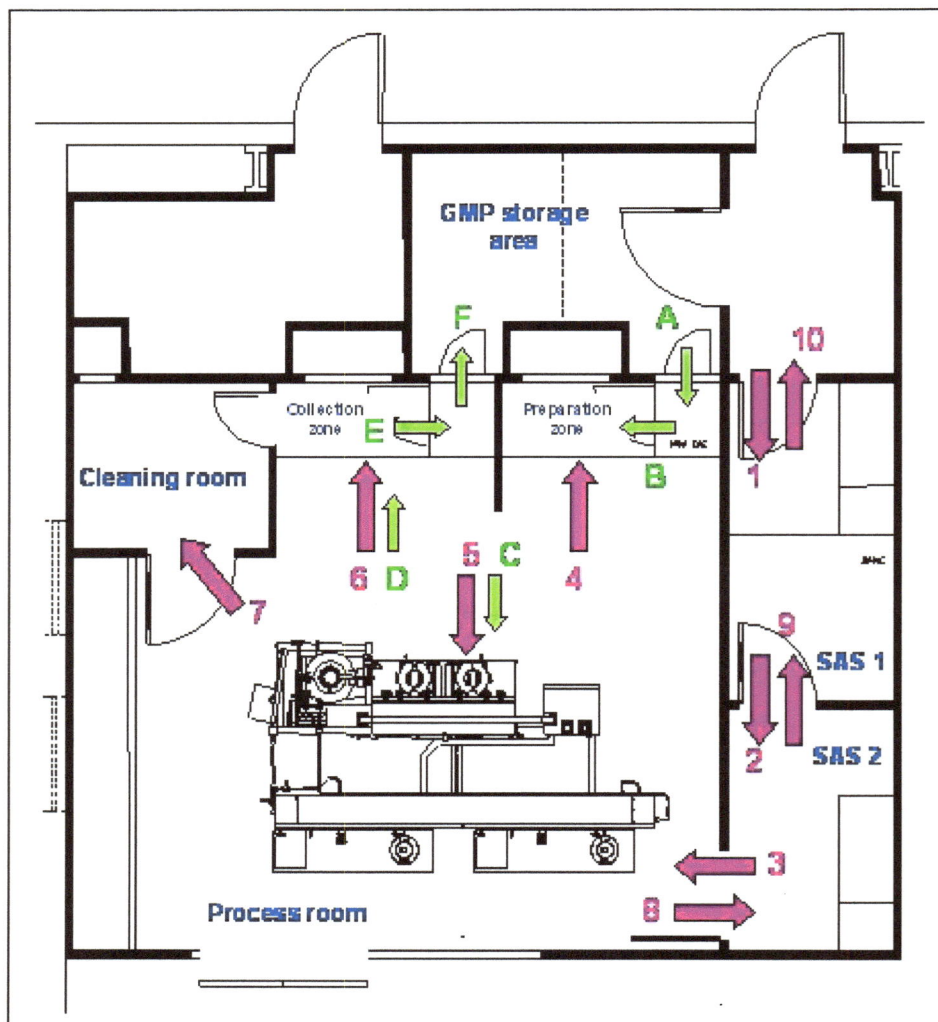

Figure 10: Clean room for GMP manufacturing of potent APIs (*Courtesy of SEPAREX*) (letter labelled dots: drug substance, figure labelled dots: operators).

In any case, the vent streams should be collected and scrubbed before venting to the atmosphere. This is mandatory to avoid any release of active drugs to the atmosphere either during normal operation or during a sudden decompression of the unit (e.g. caused by the rupture of a safety burst disk, by a leakage or by an emergency stop) which could result in the release of a powder aerosol. High pressure filters can be used in most of the normal operation venting lines. However, for the safety venting line, this solution is not adequate and it was proposed to contain, and preferably to scrub, the vent streams in a pressure vessel with an internal volume large enough to contain the whole capacity of the unit.

Scale-Up of Particle Design Processes

With the major exception of GAS and batch coating of preformed particles, all SCF particle design processes are spray-based processes. This feature is of major importance because the scale-up of such spray-based processes is complex with the following key issues: control of the particle size distribution upon scaling-up and particle collection. Numerous issues still have to be solved before successful scale-up of these techniques at a commercial scale. Beyond scale-up heuristics, reaching commercial scale with SCF spray-based processes will require to tackle issues related to many complementary areas as follows:

- better understanding of the particle generation process (supersaturation, rate of nucleation, post nucleation growth, agglomeration);

- residual solvent removal for SC anti-solvent processes;

- harvesting of micronic or submicronic particles with a high yield and under cGMP conditions.

For RESS, most of the described applications involve an expansion at atmospheric pressure, and hence the supply or recycling cost of carbon dioxide is an issue. All the more since solubility in the SCF is low in most cases and thus very large fluid to product ratios are required. Another complex issue for the scale-up of RESS is the large decrease of temperature caused by the rapid expansion of SC CO_2. Enhanced by the use of large flow rates, this cooling issue leads to a necessary large enthalpy input to prevent the formation of a liquid phase during expansion.

As pointed out earlier, starting from organic or aqueous solutions, the SC anti-solvent processes appear to be the most versatile SC processes for particle design, including the manufacturing of composite particle. The main limitation of the SCF-based anti-solvent processes remains the use of large amounts of organic solvents. Furthermore, fluid/substrate ratio of 500 up to 10,000 kg/kg are typically reported. However, in the case of a pure model substance, it was demonstrated that scale-up of an anti-solvent process can be performed from lab to commercial scale under acceptable conditions from the economical view point, with a fluid/substrate ratio as low as 50 kg/kg [84]. The elimination of residual solvent is a major concern for the production of pharmaceutical products with SCF anti-solvent processes. This step is usually carried out through direct flushing by CO_2 on the precipitated powder, leading to very high fluid/substrate ratios and, in all likelihood, to a non-homogeneous product due to channeling issue. The stripping solvent efficiency is a balance of the solute/solvent affinity with respect to its interaction with the anti-solvent. Polymers and proteins, with high affinity for the solvent, are typically difficult to wash [85,86]. It also depends on the solid arrangement of the powder, and the efficiency of percolation through the powder bed. In order to properly scale-up the anti-solvent processes, the washing step should very likely be designed and operated as a separate operation to overcome the low efficiency of solvent extraction.

The PGSS process is already used for particle design at the industrial scale for the production of powder coating formulations and paints [87] and for the manufacturing of powdered food and food derived products. A commercial scale plant, equipped with continuous powder harvesting from the spraying vessel, has been recently taken into operation for the production of up to 300 kg per hour of food products [1]. It makes a big difference with the other SC particle design processes which are still at the early (i.e. pilot) development stage at the present time, even if several projects dealing with the GMP manufacturing of clinical batches by SC anti-solvent processes and an example of deoiling of 120 kg per hour of lecithin by a SCF-antisolvent process have been reported [74]. The CO_2 consumption is low for PGSS and volumes of high-pressure vessels are smaller than those needed for RESS or anti-solvent processes. For PGSS and PGSS-related processes operated at an industrial scale of about 1,500 kg of powder per hour, it has been reported that the production cost, including investment, personal, consumables and maintenance, ranges from 0.20 € to 1 € per kg of powder depending on the annual operation time and CO_2/powder ratio [1]. According to these authors, using a CO_2 recycling loop, the cost could reach values below 0.15 € per kg of powder. The simplicity of this solvent-free process, associated with the low processing costs and the wide range of products that can be processed, should provide true opportunities for the development of PGSS at commercial scale for food and pharmaceutical applications, for instance for the manufacturing of solid dispersions of poorly soluble drugs.

From our experience, the recovery of micronic or submicronic particles of valuable and potent products with high yield and under operating conditions compliant with the pharmaceutical standards is one of the key issues for the commercial success of SCF particle design processes. Obviously, this issue becomes of major concern for the production of dry nanoparticles, which are very difficult to handle. Because of the major issue related to fine precipitate harvesting, spray-based anti-solvent processes are until now operated as batch processes as far as potent products are concerned.

The particles are trapped on filters, sintered plates or bags during the particle generation step and then collected after depressurization of the high pressure vessel. This technique often results in caking of the particles or clogging of the filters. Moreover, the collection of particles under pharmaceutical standards seems difficult to reach at a large scale and acceptable cost based on this discontinuous lab scale technical solution. At a large scale, it should be advantageous to continuously or semi-continuously withdraw the particles from the high-pressure vessel, as described for a production plant for the deoiling of raw lecithin [74], or at least to transfer by clean, automated and reproducible means a batch of precipitate to an intermediate vessel before dispatching the powder in the final dosage containers.

SCF PROCESSES AND GMP

Pharmaceutical production must be compliant with the cGMP requirements, briefly described as follows : (i) the equipment is properly designed, installed and commissioned (ii) the process is reliable and is shown to be capable of consistently manufacturing products of the required quality and complying with their specifications, with the necessary level of traceability and documentation. Therefore, prior to the production of drug products either for clinical trials or for human administration, the equipment and process should undergo an in-depth validation, including all necessary qualification steps.

Since the earlier design step, the compliance of the equipment manufacturing should take into account the restrictions regarding the nature of materials, such as stainless steel (i.e. 316L) and seals. All materials must also be supplied with a complete manufacturing record. A major feature of cGMP is also the necessity to perform an easy, efficient, reproducible and validated cleaning of the equipment. For reproducibility purposes, automated cleaning in place is preferred, and should be taken into account at the earliest stages of equipment design and manufacturing. The cleaning requirement dictates an optimisation of the design of each component in contact with the products, particularly as regards the absence of dead-volumes, low surface roughness of materials and design of easy to clean connections. The cleaning issue is strongly linked to the requirement to maintain the highest standards of

product safety, therefore to avoid the product contamination, which could either be outside contamination during processing, or cross-contamination from previously processed products. The cross-contamination is a major concern, as most of the SCF processes could find applications for low-volume high-value products, which could be processed using a multi-product plant. Some specific cross-contamination issues of SCF processes were recently discussed [8], such as the contamination from fluid recycling or from the CO_2 supply system.

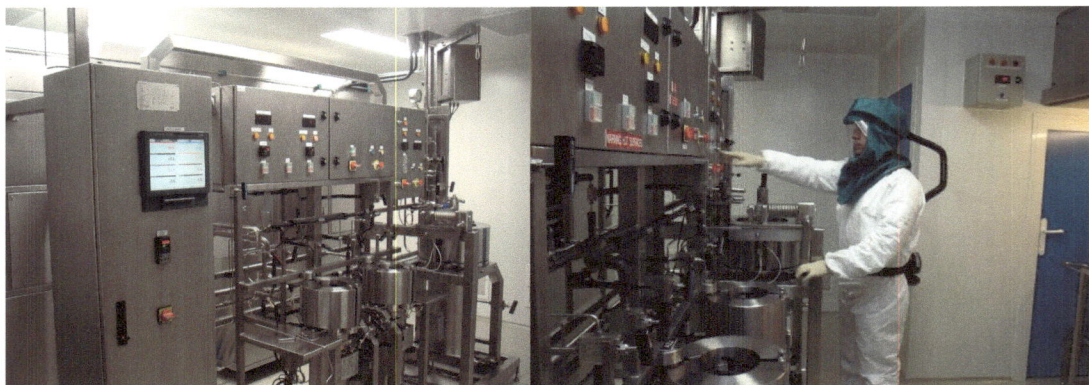

Figure 11: SCF particle design pilot GMP unit (*Courtesy of Separex*)

Most of the components of a SCF particle production unit are similar to those used for already scaled-up SCF processes such as batch extraction of natural products, continuous counter-current fluid/liquid fractionation, preparative supercritical chromatography, or production of powder coatings. As already underlined for SFE and SFF processes, the design and manufacturing of large high-pressure vessels, high-pressure pumps and valves, safety equipments and process control tools are fully mastered and many large volume high-pressure plants are currently running. The operation, safety and reliability of such high-pressure units are thus well mastered. However, most of these plants are operated under chemical or food industry standards. Hence, the technical choice of any part must be considered in order to match GMP requirements (tubing and autoclave polishing, valve lubrication, dust deposition, etc.) with a special attention to cleaning operability and subsequent consequences on hardware design. For instance, SEPAREX (France) recently built and operated a semi-industrial plant for clinical lot manufacturing (0.5 – 5 kg) of high-potent APIs as shown on Fig. **11**. In fact, the SCF particle design process itself (i.e. RESS or ASES) had to be completely reconsidered and very innovative solutions were developed. Most sections for particle collection, fluid recycle and waste management, as no effluent containing API could be rejected outside, were specifically addressed. GMP compliant instrumentation and data logging were implemented, including all environmental parameters inside the clean room where the unit is operated.

CONCLUSION

SCF-based processes have great potential for processing of food or food-related products, pure pharmaceutical materials and drug-loaded composite particles. SCF extraction and fractionation processes are now established industrial techniques with several hundred plants in operation worldwide. In addition, SCF particle design processes make it possible to address key issues of food processing and drug formulation which are related to control of particle size distribution, morphology, crystallinity and stability of solid particles. However, many efforts are still required in order to scale-up these particle engineering processes at full scale for a wider range of applications, including the GMP-compliant manufacturing of pharmaceuticals. The scale-up of SCF particle engineering processes and the design of suitable industrial equipment demand completely new approaches, especially for enthalpy supply (RESS), particle collection (when neat and dry nano- or micro-particles are required), residual solvent stripping (anti-solvent). These processes offer the possibility to produce unique products and have been extensively studied for pharmaceutical or food applications with some recent examples of manufacturing of clinical batches for pharmaceutical applications and the operation of large plant for food applications. It is hence believed that they will very likely find new applications at the industrial scale in the near future.

REFERENCES

[1]   Weidner E., *J. Supercrit. Fluids*, Vol. 47, **2009**, p 556-565
[2]   Clavier J.Y., Perrut M., In: R von Rohr, C Trepp, ed. *High Pressure Chemical Engineering*, Amsterdam: Elsevier, **1996**, p. 627
[3]   Brunner G., *J. Supercrit. Fluids*, Vol. 47, **2009**, p. 574-582
[4]   Calm J.M., Hourahan G.C., *HPAC Engineering*, Vol. 79, **2007**, p. 50-64
[5]   Catchpole O.J., Tallon S.J., Eltringham W.E., Grey J.B., Fenton K.A., Vagi E.M., Vyssotski M.V., Mackenzie A.N., Ryan J., Zhu Y., *J. Supercrit. Fluids*, Vol. 47, **2009**, p. 591-597
[6]   Clifford A. A., In Proceedings of the 9th International Symposium on Supercritical Fluids, Ecole des Mines d'Albi-Carmaux Ed., **2009**, Oral C12
[7]   Geyer S., Schulmeyr J., Gehrig M., In Proceedings of the 9th International Symposium on Supercritical Fluids, Ecole des Mines d'Albi-Carmaux Ed., **2009**, Poster P133
[8]   Clavier J.Y., Perrut M., In: P. York, U.B. Kompella, B.Y. Shekunov (Edts.), *Supercritical Fluid Technology for drug Product Development*, Vol. 18, New-York: Marcel Dekker, **2004**, p. 615
[9]   Brunner G., *Gas extraction*, Darmstadt: Steinkopff, **1994**
[10] Stahl E., Quirin K.W., Gerard D., ed. *Dense Gases for Extraction and Refining*, Berlin Heidelberg: Springer-Verlag, **1988**
[11] Diaz M.S., Brignole E.A., *J. Supercrit. Fluids*, Vol. 47, **2009**, p. 611
[12] Clavier J.Y., Majewski W., Perrut M., In: R von Rohr, C Trepp, ed. *High Pressure Chemical Engineering*, Amsterdam: Elsevier, **1996**, p. 639
[13]   Temelli F., *J. Supercrit. Fluids*, Vol. 47, **2009**, p. 583-590
[14] Lack E., Seidlitz H., Bakali M., Zobel R., In Proceedings of the 9th International Symposium on Supercritical Fluids, Ecole des Mines d'Albi-Carmaux Ed., **2009**, Oral C04
[15] Luetge C., Stainhagen V., Bork M., Knez Z., In Proceedings of the 9th International Symposium on Supercritical Fluids, Ecole des Mines d'Albi-Carmaux Ed., **2009**, Oral C05

[16] King J.W., Srinivas K., *J. Supercrit. Fluids*, Vol. 47, **2009**, p. 598-610

[17] Kompella U.B., Koushik K., *Crit. Rev. Therap. Drug Carrier Syst.*, Vol. 18, **2001**, p. 173

[18] York P., Kompella U.B., Shekunov B.Y., ed. Supercritical Fluid Technology for drug Product Development. Drugs and Pharmaceutical Sciences Vol. 18, New-York: Marcel Dekker, **2004**

[19] Jung, J., Perrut M., *J. Supercrit. Fluids*, Vol. 20, **2001**, p. 179

[20] Amidon G.L., Lennerna H., Shah V.P., Crison J.R., *Pharm. Res.*, Vol. 12, **1995**, p. 413

[21] Aungst B.J., *J. Pharm. Sci.*, Vol. 82, **1993**, p. 979

[22] Eerikainen H., Watanabe W., Kauppinen E., Ahonen P., *Eur. J. Pharm. Biopharm. Sci.*, Vol. 18, **2003**, p. 113

[23] Shoyele S.A., Cawthorne S., *Adv. Drug. Deliver. Rev.*, Vol. 58, **2006**, p.1009

[24] Serajuddin A.T.M., *J. Pharm. Sci.*, Vol. 88, **1999**, p. 1058

[25] Froemming K.H., Szejtli J., Cyclodextrins in Pharmacy, Kluwer, Dordrecht, **1994**

[26] Richard J., Deschamps F.S., In Colloidal Polymers : Preparation and Biomedical Applications, A. Elaissari (ed), Marcel Dekker, New York, **2004**, p. 429

[27] Ogawa Y., *J. Biomater. Sci. Polymer Edn*, Vol. 8, **1997**, p. 391

[28] Couvreur P., Dubernet C., Puisieux F., *Eur. J. Pharm. Biopharm.*, Vol. 41, **1995**, p. 2

[29] Maeda H., *Adv. Enzyme Regul.*, Vol. 41, **2001**, p. 89

[30] Broadhead J, Edmond Rouan S.K., Rhodes C.T., *Drug Dev. Ind. Pharm.*, Vol. 18, **1992**, p. 1169

[31] Otsuka M., Kaneniwa N., *Int. J. Pharm.*, Vol. 62, **1990**, p. 65

[32] Date A.A., Patravale V.B., *Current Opinion Colloids Interf. Sci.*, Vol. 9, **2004**, p. 222

[33] Matson D.W., Fulton J.L., Petersen R.C., Smith R.D., *Ind. Eng. Chem.Res.*, Vol. 26, **1987**, p. 2298

[34] Gallagher P.M., Coffey M.P., Krukonis V.J., *J. Supercrit. Fluids*, Vol. 5, **1992**, p. 130

[35] Bleich J., Müller B.W., *J. Microencapsulation*, Vol. 13, **1996**, p. 131

[36] Weidner E., Knez Z., Novak Z., Proc. 3rd Int. Symp. Supercrit. Fluids, Vol. 3, **1994**, p. 229

[37] Weidner E., Steiner R., Dirschel H., Weinreich B., Patent EP 9705484, **1997**

[38] Duarte A.R.C., Simplicio A.L., Vega-Gonzalez A., Subra-Paternault P., Coimbra P., Gil M.H., De Sousa H.C., *J. Supercritical Fluids*, Vol. 42, **2007**, p.373

[39] Türk M., Upper G., Steurenthaler M., Hussein Kh., Wahl M.A., *J. Supercrit. Fluids*, Vol. 39, **2007**, p. 435

[40] Chattopadhyay P., Huff R., Shekunov B.Y., *J. Pharm. Sci.*, Vol. 95, **2006**, p. 667

[41] Ventosa N., Sala S., Veciana J., *J. Supercrit. Fluids*, Vol. 26, **2003**, p. 33

[42] Richard J., Deschamps F., Thomas O., In "Polymeric Drug Delivery; Volume II: Polymeric Matrices and Drug Particle Engineering", Ed. By S. Sonke (American Chemical Society), **2006**, p. 250

[43] Verreck G., Decorte A., Heymans K., Adriaensen J., Liu D., Tomasko D.L., Arien A., Peeters J., Rombaut P., Van den Mooter G., Brewster M.E., *J. Supercrit. Fluids*, Vol. 40, **2007**, p. 153

[44] Türk M., *J. Supercritical Fluids*, Vol. 47 , **2009**, p. 537-545

[45] Tom J.W., Debenedetti PG., Jerome R., *J. Supercrit. Fluids*, Vol. 7, **1994**, p. 9

[46] Kim J.H., Paxton T.E., Tomasko D.L., *J. Supercrit. Fluids*, Vol. 7, **1996**, p. 9

[47] Türk M., Upper G., Hils P., *J. Supercritical Fluids*, Vol. 39, **2006**, p. 253-263

[48] Türk M., Hils P., Helfgen B., Schaber K., Martin H.-J., Wahl M.A., *J. Supercrit. Fluids*, Vol. 22, **2002**, p. 75

[49] Domingo C., Berends E., Van Rosmalen G.M., *J. Supercrit. Fluids*, Vol. 10, **1997**, p. 39

[50] Young T.J., Mawson S., Johnston K.P., Henriksen I.B., Pace G.W., Mishra A.K., *Biotechnol. Prog.*, Vol. 16, **2000**, p. 402

[51] Perrut M., Jung J., Leboeuf F., *Int. J. Pharmaceut.*, Vol. 288, **2005**, p. 11

[52] Perrut M., Jung J., Leboeuf F.,. *Int. J. Pharmaceut.*, Vol. 288, **2005**, p. 3

[53] Jovanovic N., Bouchard A., Hofland G.W., Witkamp G.-J., Crommelin D.J.A., Jiskoot W., *Pharm. Res.*, Vol. 21, **2004**, p. 1955

[54] Bouchard A., Jovanovic N., Jiskoot W., Mendes E., Witkamp G.J., Crommelin D.J.A, Hofland G.W., *J. Supercrit. Fluids*, Vol. 40, **2007**, p. 293

[55] Dixon D.J., Johnston K.P., Bodmeier R.A., *AIChE J.*, Vol. 39, **1993**, p. 127

[56] Müller B.W., Fischer W., Patent DE 3744329, **1989**

[57] Hanna M., York P., Patent WO 96/00610, **1995**

[58] Reverchon E., *J. Supercrit. Fluids*, Vol. 15, **1999**, p. 1

[59] Randolph T.W., Randolph A.D., Mebes M., Yeung S., *Biotechnol. Prog.*, Vol. 9, **1993**, p. 429

[60] Subramaniam B., Proceedings of the AAPS Annual Meeting, Pharm. Sci. 1, S-615, **1998**

[61] Mawson S., Kanakia S., Johnston K., *J. Appl. Polym. Sci.*, Vol. 64, **1997**, p. 2105

[62] Perrut M., Jung J., Leboeuf F., In Proceedings of the Fourth International Symposium on High Pressure Process Technology & Chemical engineering, Venice (Italy), AIDIC: Milano, **2002**, p.711

[63] Chow A.H.L., Tong H.H.Y., Shekunov B.Y., In: P York, UB Kompella, BY Shekunov, ed. Supercritical Fluid Technology for drug Product Development. Drugs and Pharmaceutical Sciences Vol. 18, New-York: Marcel Dekker, **2004**, p. 283

[64]   Moribe K., Tozuka Y., Yamamoto K., *Adv. Drug Delivery Rev.*, Vol. 60, **2008**, p. 328-338

[65]   Muhrer G., Meier U., Fusaro F., Albano S., Mazzotti M., *Int. J. Pharm.*, Vol. 308, **2006**, p. 69

[66]   Juppo A.M., Boissier C., Khoo C., *Int. J. Pharm.*, Vol. 250, **2003**, p. 385

[67]   Majerik V., Charbit G., Badens E., Horvath G., Szokonya L., Bosc N., Teillaud E., *J.Supercrit. Fluids*, Vol. 40, **2007**, p. 101

[68]   Jung J., Leboeuf F., Fabing I., Perrut M., patent WO 02/32462, **2002**

[69]   Lochard H., Rodier E., Sauceau M., Letourneau J.J., Freiss B., Joussot-Dubien C., Fages J., Proceedings of the 6th International Symposium on Supercritical Fluids, G. Brunner, I. Kikic, M. Perrut, Ed.., **2003**, p. 1659.

[70]   Rodier E., Lochard H., Sauceau M., Letourneau J.J., Freiss B., Fages J., *Eur. J. Pharm. Sci.*, Vol. 26, **2005**, p. 184

[71]   Van Hees T., Piel G., Evrard B., Otte X., Thunus L., Delattre L., *Pharm. Res.*, Vol. 16, **1999**, p. 1864

[72]   Hussein K., Türk M, Wahl M.A., *Pharm. Res.*, Vol. 24, **2007**, p. 585

[73]   Stahl E., Quirin K.W., Glatz A., Gerard D., Rau G., Ber. Bunsenges *Phys. Chem.*, Vol. 88, **1984**, p. 900

[74]   Bork M., Luetge C., Knez Z., Proceedings of the 1ˢᵗ Iberoamerican Conference on Supercritical Fluids, Igassu Falls (Brazil), April 10ᵗʰ-13ᵗʰ, **2007** – CD-ROM

[75]   Tomasko D., Li H., Liu D., Han X., Wingert M., Lee L., Koelling K.A., *Ind. Eng. Chem. Res.*, Vol. 42, **2003**, p. 6431

[76]   Tomasko D. et al., Understanding and Exploiting Tg Reduction for Surface and Bulk Modification f Polymers with CO2, 10th European Meeting on Supercritical Fluids, Colmar (France), 12-14 december **2005**

[77]   Munuklu P., Jansens P.J., *J. Supercrit. Fluids*, Vol. 40, **2007**, p. 433

[78]   De Sousa A.R.S, Calderone M., Rodier E., Fages J., Duarte C.M.M., *J. Supercrit. Fluids*, Vol.39, **2006**, p. 13

[79]   Wissinger R.G., Paulatis M.E., *J. Polym. Sci. Part B*, Vol. 29, **1991**, p. 631

[80]   Gulari E., Manke C.W., Proceedings of the 5th International Symposium on Supercritical Fluids, Atlanta (USA), **2000**.

[81]   Jung J., Leboeuf F., Perrut M., In: M Besnard, F Cansell, ed. Proceedings of the 8th Meeting on Supercritical Fluids, Bordeaux (France), **2002**, p. 805

[82]   Shine A., Gelb J., Patent WO 98/15348, **1997**

[83]   Clavier J.Y., Proceedings of the 6th international symposium on Supercritical Fluids, Versailles, Tome 3, p. 1843, **2003**

[84]   Jung J., Clavier J.Y., Perrut M., Proceedings of the 6th international symposium on Supercritical Fluids, Versailles, **2003**, p. 1683

[85]   Thiering R., Deghani F., Foster N.L., *J. Supercrit. Fluids*, Vol. 21, **2001**, p. 159

[86]   Ruchatz F., Kleinebudde P., Muller B.W., *J. Pharm. Sc.*, Vol. 86, **1997**, p. 101

[87]   Mandel F.S., Wang J.D., *Inorg. Chim. Acta*, Vol. 294, **1999**, p. 214

INDEX

A

Active compound 11, 29, 33 – 35, 52, 57, 78, 98

B

Biomaterials 6
Biopolymers 16, 23

C

CAN-BD 12, 32
Catalyst precursors 23
Chemistry 3,4
Chrastil equation 42, 86
Controlled release 8, 29, 36, 38, 52, 54, 57, 102, 108
Couloring matters 16
Crystal 16 – 18, 21, 25, 61, 104, 107
Crystallization 8, 25, 30, 53, 61, 103
Cyclodextrin 11, 20, 22, 34, 102, 108

D

DELOS 12, 33, 34, 103
Density 2, 42, 46, 47, 62-66, 85
Desorption model 8, 87, 89, 90
Diffusion model 88, 89
Drug delivery 8, 9, 14, 38, 52, 54, 56, 59, 102, 103

E

Encapsulation 6, 9, 37, 37, 88, 108, 109
Enzyme 22, 34
Equation of State (EOS) 24, 41-45, 67, 87
Explosives 16, 23
Extraction 1, 3, 4, 61, 66, 71-79, 80-96, 97, 99, 100-102

F

Fractionation 2,3, 71-79, 97-102
Fugacity 42

G

Gas Anti-solvent (GAS) 5, 17, 46, 103, 106, 111
GMP 14, 38, 97, 110-112
GRAS 2, 3
Group Contribution (GC) EOS 43

I

Impregnation 4, 9, 52-60, 103
Industrial scale 5, 11, 14, 71, 74, 91, 92, 97, 99, 110 -113
Industry 1, , 6, 9, 30, 53, 62, 68, 97, 102, 109
Ionic liquid 5, 61-70

L

Lipid 8, 11, 13, 34-38, 45, 53, 71, 100, 102, 103, 108, 109
Liposomes 8

M

Mass transfer 5, 14, 16, 21, 24, 25, 32, 41, 48, 53, 62, 67, 77, 80-96, 107

Mathematical modelling 16, 41, 43, 44, 49, 80-96
Micronization 8, 16- 28, 97, 102, 103
Microparticles 16-28, 59, 105, 107
Miscibility switch 61, 66-68
Molar volume 46, 66
Molecular imprinting 54

N
Nanoparticles 5, 8, 9, 16 – 28, 31, 53, 103, 108, 112
Natural products 2, 3, 13, 80, 98, 101, 113
Nucleation 12, 24-26, 31, 44, 104, 107, 111
Nutraceutical 36, 97, 102, 104

P
Particle coating 9, 12, 33
Particle engineering 6, 29, 97, 98, 102, 103
Particle formation 6, 8, 9, 14, 25, 34, 41, 45, 49, 53, 97, 102-106
Particle Gas Saturated Solutions (PGSS) 5, 13, 29-40, 44, 45, 104, 108, 109, 111, 112
Peng-Robinson EOS 42, 43
Perturbed Hard-Sphere-Chain (PHSC) EOS 43
Pharmaceutical 6, 8, 9, 11, 14, 19, 34, 35, 52-54, 60,65, 68, 97, 102, 103, 109-112
Phase behaviour 14, 67, 75, 90
Phase diagram 16, 24, 46, 64, 67, 68
Phase equilibrium 5, 43, 46, 47, 49, 68, 74, 75, 79, 80, 82, 85, 90, 92
Polymer 4, 6, 8, 10, 12, 13, 16, 23, 34, 43, 53-60
Polymerization 9, 58
Precipitation 6, 8-15, 16-28, 41-51, 53, 104, 108
Protein 13, 22, 34, 48, 103, 106, 111

R
Rapid Expansion Supercritical Solution (RESS) 9 -11, 43, 45, 103 – 106, 111
Reaction 4, 5, 61-70
RESOLV (Rapid Expansion of Supercritical Solutions into a liquid solvent) 12

S
Safety 8, 14, 55, 60, 63, 69, 97-99, 100, 113
Sanchez-Lacombe EOS 43
Scaffolds 6
Scale-up 10, 14, 30, 41, 80, 81, 92, 97, 99-102, 104, 111-113
Shrinking core model 88, 91
Solubility 5, 10-12, 35, 41-46, 53, 55, 59, 62, 63, 65, 66, 68, 73, 75-77, 85-88, 100, 102, 105, 106, 111
Statistical Associating Fluid Theory (SAFT) EOS 43
Superconductor precursors 19, 22, 23
Supercritical Anti-solvent 5, 9, 16-28, 54, 55, 103, 106, 111
Supercritical Assisted Atomization (SAA) 32
Supercritical Fluid Extraction of Emulsions (SFEE) 103
Supercritical water 1-5
Supersaturation 5, 25, 41, 43, 103, 104, 106, 111
Swelling 6, 44, 48, 53, 104, 109, 110

V
Viscosity 5, 21, 30, 44, 62, 63, 64, 87, 103, 106, 108

W
Weber number 21, 25, 43, 44

www.ingramcontent.com/pod-product-compliance
Lightning Source LLC
Chambersburg PA
CBHW041718210326
41598CB00007B/697